New Psychoactive Substances

New Psychoactive Substances

Edited by

KRISTINA ADORJAN

Director and Full Professor,
Department of Psychiatry and Psychotherapy (UPD),
University of Bern, Switzerland

Director of Teaching and Research (UPD),
University of Bern, Switzerland

Vice Dean for Internationalization and National Networking,
Faculty of Medicine, University of Bern, Switzerland

THOMAS G. SCHULZE

Professor, LMU Munich, Bavaria, Germany and
SUNY Upstate Medical University, Syracuse, New York, USA;
President-Elect, World Psychiatric Association (WPA);
Member, German National Academy of Sciences Leopoldin

SHARON L. WALSH

Professor of Behavioral Science, Pharmacology,
Pharmaceutical Sciences and Psychiatry,
University of Kentucky Colleges of Medicine and Pharmacy,
Lexington, Kentucky, USA

OXFORD
UNIVERSITY PRESS

OXFORD
UNIVERSITY PRESS

Oxford University Press is a department of the University of Oxford.
It furthers the University's objective of excellence in research, scholarship,
and education by publishing worldwide. Oxford is a registered trade mark of
Oxford University Press in the UK and in certain other countries.

Published in the United States of America by Oxford University Press
198 Madison Avenue, New York, NY 10016, United States of America.

Library of Congress Cataloging-in-Publication Data
Names: Adorjan, Kristina editor | Schulze, Thomas G. editor |
Walsh, Sharon (Sharon L.) editor
Title: New psychoactive substances / [edited by] Kristina Adorjan,
Thomas G. Schulze, and Sharon L. Walsh.
Description: New York : Oxford University Press, [2026] |
Includes bibliographical references.
Identifiers: LCCN 2025048808 (print) | LCCN 2025048809 (ebook) |
ISBN 9780190095697 paperback | ISBN 9780190095703 ebook |
ISBN 9780190095710 epub | ISBN 9780190095727 Digital Online
Subjects: LCSH: Psychotropic drugs | Psychotropic drugs—Physiological effect |
Psychotropic drugs—Side effects | Psychotropic drugs—Law and legislation | Drug abuse
Classification: LCC RM315 .N494 2026 (print) | LCC RM315 (ebook)
LC record available at https://lccn.loc.gov/2025048808
LC ebook record available at https://lccn.loc.gov/2025048809

DOI: 10.1093/med/9780190095697.001.0001

Printed by Marquis Book Printing, Canada

The manufacturer's authorized representative in the EU for product safety is
Oxford University Press España S.A. of Parque Empresarial San Fernando de Henares,
Avenida de Castilla, 2 – 28830 Madrid (www.oup.es/en or product.safety@oup.com).
OUP España S.A. also acts as importer into Spain of products made by the manufacturer.

FSC www.fsc.org MIX Paper | Supporting responsible forestry FSC® C103567

Contents

Contributors

Sophia Achab, Director, WHOCC, Geneva University and Clinical Director ReConnecte Specialized Treatment Centre, University Hospitals of Geneva

Kristina Adorjan, Director and Full Professor, Department of Psychiatry and Psychotherapy (UPD), University of Bern, Switzerland; Director of Teaching and Research (UPD), University of Bern, Switzerland; Vice Dean for Internationalization and National Networking, Faculty of Medicine, University of Bern, Switzerland

Davide Arillotta, Department of Pharmacology, University of Florence, Italy; Psychopharmacology, Drug Misuse & Novel Psychoactive Substances Research Unit, School of Life & Medical Sciences, University of Hertfordshire, College Lane Campus, Hatfield, United Kingdom

Alexander Baldacchino, Professor of Medicine, Psychiatry and Addiction, University of St Andrews Medical School, North Haugh, St Andrews, Fife, Scotland

Giuseppe Bersani, Department of Clinical, Pharmacological and Biological Sciences, College Lane, University of Hertfordshire, Hatfield, United Kingdom; Department of Medico-Surgical Sciences and Biotechnologies, Sapienza University of Rome, Italy

Roshan Bhad, Additional Professor of Psychiatry, National Drug Dependence Treatment Centre (NDDTC), All India Institute of Medical Sciences (AIIMS), New Delhi, India

Tobias Bracht, Head of the Competence Center for Interventional Psychiatry and Augmented Psychotherapy, Research Group Leader, University Hospital of Psychiatry, Bern, Switzerland

Valeria Catalani, Psychopharmacology, Drug Misuse & Novel Psychoactive Substances Research Unit, School of Life & Medical Sciences, University of Hertfordshire, College Lane Campus, Hatfield, United Kingdom

Stefania Chiappini, Psychopharmacology, Drug Misuse & Novel Psychoactive Substances Research Unit, School of Life & Medical Sciences, University of Hertfordshire, College Lane Campus, Hatfield, United Kingdom

Ornella Corazza, School of Medicine, Hertfordshire University, United Kingdom; Addiction Science Lab, University of Trento

John Martin Corkery, Psychopharmacology, Drug Misuse & Novel Psychoactive Substances Research Unit, School of Life & Medical Sciences, University of Hertfordshire, College Lane Campus, Hatfield, United Kingdom

Niklaus Denier, Senior Physician at the Competence Center for Interventional Psychiatry and Augmented Psychotherapy, Researcher, University Hospital of Psychiatry Bern, Switzerland

Hamed Ekhtiari, Director of Neuroscience-Informed Interventions for Addiction Medicine (NIAM) Lab, Laureate Institute for Brain Research, Tulsa, Oklahoma; Medical Discovery Team on Addiction (MDTA), University of Minnesota

Hussien Elkholy, Clinical Assistant Professor in Psychiatry, Department of Clinical Neuroscience, Brighton and Sussex Medical School, United Kingdom; Professor of Psychiatry, Department of Neurology and Psychiatry, Faculty of Medicine, Ain Shams University, Cairo, Egypt

Jürg Gertsch, Institute of Biochemistry and Molecular Medicine (IBMM), University of Bern, Switzerland

Katharina Elisabeth Grafinger, Institute of Forensic Medicine, Forensic Toxicology and Chemistry, University of Bern, Switzerland

Amira Guirguis, Swansea University Medical School, Institute of Life Sciences 2, Swansea University, Singleton Park, Swansea, United Kingdom

Rama Kamal, Director Research and Education, Senior Consultant Psychiatrist and Senior Consultant Addiction Medicine, Doha, Qatar

Sara L. Kroll, Social and Affective Neuropsychopharmacology, Adult Psychiatry and Psychotherapy, University Hospital of Psychiatry Zurich, University of Zurich, Switzerland

Katarzyna Kuczyńska, Department of Pharmacodynamics, Medical University of Lodz, Poland

Felix Müller, Head of the Research Group for Substance-Assisted Therapy, University Hospital of Psychiatry Basel, Switzerland

Philippe Pfeifer, Head of the Research Group for Substance-Assisted Therapy, University Hospital of Psychiatry and Psychotherapy, Bern, Switzerland

Elisabeth Prevete, Psychiatry and Clinical Psychopharmacology University Unit, ASL Latina Hospital, Terracina, Italy

Boris B. Quednow, Experimental Pharmacopsychology and Psychological Addiction Research, Adult Psychiatry and Psychotherapy, University Hospital of Psychiatry Zurich, University of Zurich, Switzerland

Norbert Scherbaum, University of Duisburg Essen; Department of Psychiatry and Psychotherapy, Essen, Germany

Fabrizio Schifano, Psychopharmacology, Drug Misuse & Novel Psychoactive Substances Research Unit, School of Life & Medical Sciences, University of Hertfordshire, College Lane Campus, Hatfield, United Kingdom

Vinzenz K. Schmid, Social and Affective Neuropsychopharmacology, Adult Psychiatry and Psychotherapy, University Hospital of Psychiatry Zurich, University of Zurich, Switzerland

Yasmin Schmid, University Hospital Basel, Division of Clinical Pharmacology and Toxicology, Basel, Switzerland

Christian G. Schütz, Professor of Psychiatry, University of British Columbia, Division Head Substance Use and Concurrent Disorders, Clinician Researcher Djavad Mowafaghian Centre for Brain Health, Scientific Director Adult Mental Health and Substance Use, Provincial Health Service Authority, British Columbia, Canada

Thomas G. Schulze, Professor, LMU Munich, Bavaria, Germany, and State University of New York Upstate Medical University, Syracuse, New York, United States; President-Elect, World Psychiatric Association (WPA); Member, German National Academy of Sciences Leopoldin

Kristiana Siste, Department of Psychiatry, Dr. Cipto Mangunkusumo National Central General Hospital; Faculty of Medicine, Universitas Indonesia

Leila M. Soravia, Deputy Chief Psychologist, Research Group Leader, University Hospital of Psychiatry Bern, Switzerland

Alessandro Vento, Department of Mental Health, Rome, Italy; Addictions' Observatory (ODDPSS), Rome, Italy; Guglielmo Marconi University, Department of Psychology, Rome, Italy

Sharon L. Walsh, Professor of Behavioral Science, Pharmacology, Pharmaceutical Sciences and Psychiatry, University of Kentucky Colleges of Medicine and Pharmacy, Lexington, Kentucky, United States

Jolanta B. Zawilska, Professor Emeritus, Department of Pharmacodynamics, Medical University of Lodz, Poland

Introduction

Kristina Adorjan, Sharon L. Walsh, and Thomas G. Schulze

New psychoactive substances (NPS), often referred to as "designer drugs," "legal highs," or "research chemicals," encompass a diverse array of synthetic or semi-synthetic compounds designed to mimic or enhance the effects of traditional illicit substances, such as cannabis, cocaine, and LSD (lysergic acid diethylamide). These substances can be molecular modifications of known illegal drugs or entirely novel chemical entities. Between 2009 and 2023, the United Nations Office on Drugs and Crime (UNODC) Early Warning Advisory (EWA) documented the emergence of 1250 unique NPS across 139 countries and territories. In 2023, the number of unique NPS reported annually reached 627—the highest ever recorded in a single year.[1] Also, the diversity within the NPS market has intensified. Notably, synthetic opioids, particularly nitazenes, have emerged as a significant concern. In 2023, nitazenes accounted for 6 of the 44 new substances reported, with 16 distinct nitazenes detected globally, up from 11 in 2022. These potent opioids have been associated with a surge in overdose deaths in regions such as Estonia, Latvia, Ireland, and France.[2,3]

Concurrently, the synthetic cannabinoid market has seen unprecedented growth, with 191 unique synthetic cannabinoids reported in 2023—the highest number recorded in a single year.[4] This surge includes a significant increase in "semi-synthetic" cannabinoids, which are chemically engineered to mimic the effects of natural cannabinoids like tetrahydrocannabinol (THC). These substances often evade legal controls due to their novel chemical structures, posing challenges for detection and regulation.

The stimulant category remains the most prevalent among NPS, comprising 35% of all substances reported up to 2023.[1] This group includes synthetic cathinones and other amphetamine-like compounds, which continue to evolve rapidly, complicating enforcement and public health responses.

The rapid proliferation and chemical innovation within the NPS market present significant challenges for public health systems, regulators, law enforcement, and policymakers. The ongoing emergence of novel substances necessitates continuous monitoring, advanced forensic capabilities, and adaptive regulatory frameworks to mitigate the associated health risks and societal impacts.

Those who use or misuse NPS can suffer physical and psychological consequences, and few studies have examined these sequalae. Due to the rapid change in the compound and synthesis of substances and the continued introduction of novel chemical entities, the effects of NPS on the body can be estimated only to a limited extent. Acute intoxication is often accompanied by vegetative side effects, such as increased blood pressure, increased heart rate, chest pain, stomach and intestinal complaints, increased body temperature, heavy sweating, and increased muscle tone. Sleep disorders, anxiety, agitation, hallucinations, and seizures can also occur. Overdose or a combination with other substances can be fatal. Repeated use often leads to abuse, addiction, mental illnesses such as depression and psychosis, health problems in the physical sphere, and impairments in the quality of life. Due to permanent changes in the chemical structures of existing substances, legal controls and the detectability of NPS are only possible to a limited extent. In terms of identification, control, prevention, and treatment alternatives, NPS represent a major challenge for medicine and politics.

Based on the latest findings from science and practice in addiction medicine, this *Handbook* conveys both the basics and specialist knowledge about NPS, not only from a pharmacological and medical perspective, but also with regard to social, economic, and legal aspects. As a real practice book, the work also conveys all psychiatric and addiction medicine aspects of consumption and intoxication with NPS, including questions of prevention, comorbidity, and practical issues such as treatment approaches.

References

1. UNODC Early Warning Advisory on New Psychoactive Substances. Report 2024. 2024. https://www.unodc.org/LSS/Announcement/Details/62d5bf6f-d71e-4815-b23c-ab06b0ddd8b9?utm_source=chatgpt.com.
2. European Monitoring Centre for Drugs and Drug Addiction. European Drug Report 2024: Trends and Developments. 2024. https://www.euda.europa.eu/publications/european-drug-report/2024_en.

3. UNODC Laboratory and Scientific Service Portals. February 2024 – UNODC EWA: Nitazenes – a new group of synthetic opioids emerges. 2024. https://www.unodc.org/LSS/Announcement/Details/cbec8f4c-73aa-49ee-9e2b-75620af8a910.
4. UNODC United Nations Office on Drugs and Crime. Beyond plants: semi-synthetics diversify the cannabis market. May 2024. https://www.unodc.org/documents/scientific/SMART_Forensic_update_Vol.1.pdf.

1

New Psychoactive Substances

Definition and Classification

Katarzyna Kuczyńska and Jolanta B. Zawilska

1.1. Definition and Concepts of New Psychoactive Substances (NPS)

Over the past two decades we have witnessed a major transformation of the illicit drug market, induced by a rapid increase in the appearance and use of new psychoactive substances (NPS) with chemical structures or pharmacological profiles that are similar to traditional drugs of abuse. Generally, NPS are designed to be perceived as legal substitutes of scheduled compounds. Importantly, the illicit drug market is highly dynamic. Once a compound becomes prohibited, new unscheduled molecules quickly appear, enlarging the library of psychoactive compounds.[1–4]

The legal term for newly emerging drugs was coined by the European Union in May 2005. It defines a new psychoactive substance as a new narcotic or psychotropic drug, in pure form or in preparation, that is not scheduled under the Single Convention on Narcotic Drugs of 1961 or the Convention on Psychotropic Substances of 1971, but which may pose a public health threat comparable to that posed by substances listed in those conventions.[5] The term was adopted by the European Monitoring Centre for Drugs and Drug Addiction (EMCDDA), and a similar definition was provided by the United Nations Office on Drugs and Crime (UNODC).[2] Nevertheless, the scope of definition and legality of particular substances can vary among countries.

The term "new" may be somewhat misleading, as it suggests that compounds under consideration are newly designed or isolated. In fact, it refers to any drug that has become newly misused, including compounds invented many years ago, modified progenitors or plant-derived substances which spread beyond their natural area of occurrence. Plentiful NPS were conceived decades ago by pharmaceutical industries or universities' research staff in search of new therapeutic agents, while some of them were created to serve for research purposes exclusively (e.g., as ligands binding to distinct biological structures, mainly receptors).[2] Moreover, a few NPS are legal medicines in some countries.[6]

Today, physical and geographical boundaries do not restrict communication. Anyone can access electronic databases that contain numerous scientific sources in medicinal chemistry and pharmacology, such as articles or patents describing abandoned candidate therapeutics. Although such compounds produce unfavorable side effects and have failed registration as medicines, their documented psychoactive properties make them attractive to illegal manufacturers and consumers.[7]

Thanks to adroit strategies, NPS are offered as an alternative to controlled drugs of abuse. They can often be produced cheaply and rapidly anywhere there is access to the necessary precursor chemicals. NPS can be categorized as chemical analogues or mimetics of classical drugs of abuse and occasionally as licensed medicines. Chemical analogues share the same core structure with parent compounds but with slight modification (i.e., different constituents). However, some analogues, despite marked structural similarity, may substantially differ pharmacologically from the original compounds. On the other hand, mimetics produce the same pharmacological effects as corresponding drugs of abuse by acting on the same receptor(s) despite obvious difference in their chemical structures.[2]

1.2. Origins of the NPS Wave

The first growth in popularity of NPS dates back to the late 1970s in California (U.S.), with the appearance of new potent fentanyl analogues, α-methylfentanyl and later 3-methylfentanyl, as replacements or adulterants of heroin. At that time heroin was hardly available, was of low purity, and was expensive due to a shortage of *Papaver sommniferum* (a source of opium), planted in Afghanistan, affected by a civil war. New fentanyls were synthesized in Asia and sold under names of "China white," "China girl," or "Persian white."[8] At that time, however, NPS abuse had a limited significance to drug policy on a worldwide scale and only a few compounds were identified for the first time each year. The unprecedented irruption of NPS took place in the first decade of the twenty-first century in relation to decreasing production and purity of 3,4-methylenedioxymethamphetamine (MDMA, "ecstasy") caused by a strengthened control on the drug itself and its main precursor. Hence, new psychostimulants, such as 1-benzylpiperazine and in particular synthetic cathinones, namely methylone and mephedrone, were initially sold as MDMA or amphetamine, then were promoted as a new type of "ecstasy," and finally were sold extensively through an open market, beginning the era of "legal highs." Moreover, some psychostimulants, like mephedrone, do not serve as temporary substitutes for established controlled drugs, but persist on the market, gaining their own recognition among abusers.[1,7] As NPS do not cross-react with commercially available colorimetric methods or immunoassays, they cannot be detected by classical tests used for screening of narcotics. All NPS present in samples can only be identified by relatively costly and not widely available methods, such as gas and liquid chromatography with mass spectrometry or high-resolution mass spectrometry.[9]

1.3. Classification of NPS

NPS make up a fast-evolving, inhomogeneous group, consisting of a variety of substances. There are multiple ways to categorize NPS. For example, they can be grouped according to their origin (whether plant-based, semisynthetic, or synthetic); psychotropic effects they evoke; chemical structure; legitimacy of use; or position on the drug market.[9]

Based on exerted psychotropic effects and behavioral changes in individuals being under influence of specific substances, NPS can be organized into the following main categories:[6,10]

- *Synthetic cannabinoids*: synthetic agonists of cannabinoid receptors, mimicking the effects of Δ^9-THC, the main psychoactive ingredient of cannabis;
- *Psychostimulants*: substitutes for amphetamine, cocaine, or MDMA;
- *Hallucinogens*: exerting similar effects to LSD (lysergic acid diethylamide) or phencyclidine;
- *Depressants*: synthetic opioids (copying effects of morphine/heroin) and designer non-pharmaceutical benzodiazepines.

There is also a broad category of other compounds/substances that cannot be simply classified in the above-mentioned groups. Additionally, some diverted and misused medicines, like nitrous oxide or oxycodone, are not widely considered as NPS, although they meet the definition of NPS and their trade is not internationally controlled.[9,10] The detailed classification of NPS, with prominent representatives of each class, is provided in Table 1.1.

Synthetic cannabinoids (synthetic agonists of cannabinoid receptors, synthetic cannabinomimetics) comprise a structurally diverse group of compounds, including classical cannabinoids, family of JWH compounds named from initials of John William Huffman who first synthesized new cannabinoids (naphthoylindoles, naphtylmethylindoles, naphtoylpyrroles, naphthylmethylindenes, phenacetylindoles), acylindoles, adamantylindoles, aminoalkylindoles, benzoylindoles, cyclohexylphenols, gamma-carboline derivatives, indazoles, OXIZIDs (compounds with OXoIndoline core attached to an aZIDe linker), and TMCP compounds containing a tetramethylcyclopropane moiety (Figure 1.1). Only HU-210, which represents classical cannabinoids, shares the same chemical structure with Δ^9-tetrahydrocannabinol (Δ^9-THC), a phytocannabinoid naturally occurring in cannabis.[11]

Synthetic and recently identified on the drug market semisynthetic cannabinoids (hexahydrocannabinol, hexahydrocannabiphorol, tetrahydrocannabidiol, tetrahydrocannabiphorol, and hexahydrocannabihexol)[1] are lipophilic compounds sold as solids or oils, volatizing easily when smoked. Therefore, they are usually applied by spraying, soaking, or even sprinkling in crystalline form on a dried herbal material imitating marijuana. Recently, they have also been offered in the form of e-liquids or impregnated papers. Synthetic cannabinoids exert their pharmacological effects by activation of CB1 and CB2 cannabinoid receptors. Unlike Δ^9-THC, which is a partial agonist of these receptors, the vast majority of synthetic cannabinoids show higher affinity and efficacy at the CB1 receptor, stimulation of which is responsible for psychotropic effects. The pharmacokinetic features, such as a faster onset of effects that rapidly peaks but lasts shorter when compared to cannabis, contribute to a high abuse potential of synthetic cannabinoids. This class of NPS is used to experience marijuana-like effects, including euphoria, relaxation, disinhibition, easy laughter, and distortion of time and perception. However, they can also induce opposite psychopharmacological effects from the desired ones, such as confusion, anxiety and fear, panic attacks, psychotic episodes,

Table 1.1 Main Groups of Synthetic NPS Monitored by EMCDDA at the End of 2023[1]

Chemical Group	Representatives	Number of Compounds Monitored by EMCDDA	Psychopharmacological Activity
Synthetic cannabinoids			
JWH compounds: Naphthoylindoles Naphtylmethylindoles Naphtoylpyrroles Naphthylmethylindenes Phenacetylindoles	 JWH-018, JWH-122, JWH-073, JWH-210 JWH-175 JWH-147, JWH-145, AM-2201 JWH-176 JWH-203, JWH-250, JWH-253	254	Marijuana-like (Δ^9-THC-like)
Acylindoles	AB-005, UR-144, 5F-UR-144 (XLR-11), XLR-12		
Adamantylindoles	AB-001, APICA		
Aminoalkylindoles	WIN 55,212-2		
Benzoylindoles	AM-694, AM-2201, AM-679, RCS-4		
Cyclohexylphenols	CP 47,497		
Classical cannabinoids (dibenzopyrans)	HU-210 Hexahydrocannabihexol (HHCH), Tetrahydrocannabiphorol (THCP)		
Gamma-carboline derivatives	5F-CUMYL-PEGACLONE		
Indazoles	AKB-48 (PINACA), ADB-PINACA, MDMB-CHMICA, MDMB-BINACA, AB-FUBINACA, ADMB-3TMS-PRINACA, CUMYL-3TMS-PRINACA		

OXIZIDs	BZO-HEXOXIZID (MDA-19), BZO-POXIZID (5C-MDA-19), 5F-BZO-POXIZID (5F-MDA-19), BZO-CHMOXIZID		
TMCP compounds	TMCP-H, TMCP-018, TMCP-2201, TMCP-200, TMCP-1220		
Other	PB-22, BB-22 (QUCHIC)		
	Synthetic cathinones		
Methcathinones	Mephedrone (4-MMC), methylone, butylone (βk-MBDB), ethylone (MDEC), *N*-ethylhexedrone, *N*-ethylnorpentedrone, metaphedrone (3-MMC), 3,4-dimethylmethcathinone, (3,4-DMMC), 4-methylethcathinone, (4-MEC), 3-chloromethcathinone, (3-CMC), clephedrone (4-CMC), 3-fluoromethcathinone (3-FMC), flephedrone (4-FMC)	167	Psychostimulatory, entactogenic
α-pyrrolidinophenones (pyrovalerones)	3,4-methylenodioxypyrovalerone (MDPV), 3′,4′-methylenedioxy-α-pyrrolidinobutiophenone (3,4-MDPBP), α-pyrovalerone (α-PVP), 4-methoxy-α -pyrrolidinopentiophenone (4-MeO-PVP), α-pyrrolidinobutiophenone (α-PBP), α-pyrrolidinopropiophenone (α-PPP), 4′-methyl-α-pyrrolidinopropiophenone (MPPP), α-pyrrolidinohexanophenone (α-PHP), α- pyrrolidinoizohexanophenone (α-PiHP), α-pyrrolidinoheptanophenone (α-PHPP), 3′-methyl-α-pyrrolidinopentiophenone (3′-Me-PVP)		Psychostimulatory

(*continued*)

Table 1.1 Continued

Chemical Group	Representatives	Number of Compounds Monitored by EMCDDA	Psychopharmacological Activity
	Phenethylamines		
2C-agents (2-dimethoxyphenethylamines)	2,5-dimethoxy-4-bromophenethylamine (2C-B), 2,5- dimethoxy-4-chlorophenethylamine (2C-C), 2,5-dimethoxy-4-ethylphenethylamine (2C-E), 2,5-dimethoxy-4-iodophenethylamine (2C-I), 2,5-dimethoxy-4-propylphenethylamine (2C-P), 2,5-dimethoxy-4-methylsulfanylphenethylamine (2C-T) 2,5-dimethoxy-4-propylthiophenethylamine (2C-T-7),	93	Hallucinogenic (psychedelic)
2-D agents (2,5-dimethoxyamphetamines, DOX)	2,5-dimethoxy-4-bromoamphetamine (DOB), 2,5-dimethoxy-4-chloroamphetamine (DOC) 2,5-dimethoxy-4-methylamphetamine (DOM)		
FLY compounds	Bromo-dragonFLY, 2C-B-FLY, 2-C-B-dragonFLY, DOB-FLY		
NBOMe (N-methoxybenzyl)-2,5-dimethoxyphenethylamines	4-bromo-*N*-(methoxybenzyl)-2,5-dimethoxyphenethylamine (25B-NBOMe) 4-chloro-*N*-(methoxybenzyl)-2,5-dimethoxyphenethylamine (25C-NBOMe) 4-iodo-*N*-(methoxybenzyl)-2,5-dimethoxyphenethylamine (25I-NBOMe)		
Benzofurans Other compounds	5-(2-aminopropyl)benzofuran (5-APB), 6-(2-aminopropyl)benzofuran (6-APB), 5-(2-aminopropyl) indole (5-IT), 1-(benzofuran-5-yl)-*N*-methylpropan-2-amine (5-MAPB)	42	Hallucinogenic (psychedelic)

Opioids			
Fentanyl analogues	Acetylfentanyl, butyrylfentanyl, carfentanil, cyklopropylfentanyl, fentanyl, furanylfentanyl, *para*-fluoroisobutyrylfentanyl, remifentanil, sufentanil	81	Mimicking effects of morphine and heroine
Benzamide and 2-phenylacetamide opioids (U-compounds)	AH-7921, U-47700, *N*-ethyl-U-47700, 3,4-methylenodioxy-U-47700, U-47931E (bromadoline), U-48800, U-49900, U-50488, U-51754		
2-Benzylbenzimidazoles (nitazenes)	Etazene, etomethazene, etonitazene, *N*-desethyl etonitazene etonitazepyne (*N*-pyrrolidino etonitazene), ethyleneoxynitazene, isotonitazene, *N*-desethyl isotonitazene, metonitazene, metonitazepyne (*N*-pyrrolidino metonitazene), protonitazene,		
Other opioids	brorphine, MT-45		
Tryptamines			
Simple tryptamines: Without modification of the indole ring With modification at the 4-position on the indole ring With modification at the 5-position on the indole ring With modification at the 6-position on the indole ring	α-ethyltryptamine (AET), α-methyltryptamine (AMT), diisopropyltryptamine (DiPT) 4-acetoxy-*N,N*-diethyltryptamine (4-acetoxy-DET) 5-methoxy-*N,N*-dimethyltryptamine (5-MeO-DMT), 5-methoxy-*N*-methyl-*N*-isopropyltryptamine (5-MeO-MiPT), 5-methoxy-*N,N*-diisopropyltryptamine (5-MeO-DiPT) 6-fluoro-*N,N*-dimethyltryptamine (6-fluoro-DMT)	47	Hallucinogenic (psychedelic)
Lysergamides	2,4-dimethylazetidide (LSZ), 1-propionyl-D-lysergic acid diethylamine (1P-LSD), lysergic acid amide (LSA), 1-acetyl-lysergic acid diethylamide (ALD-52), 6-ethyl-6-nor-lysergic acid diethylamide (ETH-LAD)		

(*continued*)

Table 1.1 Continued

Chemical Group	Representatives	Number of Compounds Monitored by EMCDDA	Psychopharmacological Activity
	Benzodiazepines		
1,4-Benzodiazepines	Clonitrazepam, desmethylflunitrazepam (norflunitrazepam, fonazepam), diclazepam (2-chlorodiazepam), flubromazepam, meclozepam, nifoxipam, nitemazepam, phenazepam	36	Sedative, hypnotic
Triazolobenzodiazepines	Adinazolam, bromazolam, clonazolam, flualprazolam, flubromazolam, flunitrazolam, pyrazolam, zapizolam		
Thienotriazolobenzodiazepines	Etizolam, metizolam, fluclotizolam		
	Arylcyclohexylamines		
Methoxetamine (MXE), 2-methoxyketamine (2-MK), 3-methoxyphencyclidine (3-MeO-PCP), 4-methoxyphencyclidine (4-MeO-PCP)		27	Hallucinogenic (dissociative)
	Piperazines		
1-benzylpiperazine (BZP), 1-(3,4-methylenedioxybenzyl)piperazine (MDBZP), *meta*-chlorophenylpiperazine (mCPP)), *para*-methoxyphenylpiperazine (MeOPP), *para*-fluorophenylpiperazine (pFPP), 3-trifluoromethylphenylpiperazine (TFMPP)		16	Psychostimulatory
	Piperidines and pyrrolidines		
Desoxypipradol (2-DPMP), diphenylprolinol (D2PM)		15	Psychostimulatory
	Aminoindanes		
2-aminoindane (2-AI), *N*-methyl-2-aminoindane (*N*-methyl-2-AI), 5-iodo-2-aminoindane (5-IAI), 5-methoxy-6-methyl-2-aminoindane (MMAI), 5,6-methylenodioxy-2-aminoindane (MDAI), 5,6-methylenodioxy-*N*-methyl-2-aminoindane (MDAII)		5	Psychostimulatory

Other compounds			
Substituted amphetamines	*N*-methyl-1-(1,3-benzodioxol- 5-yl)-2-butanamine) (MBDB), 3,4-methylenedioxy-*N,N*-dimethylamphetamine (MDDM), *para*-methoxyamphetamine (PMA), *para*-methoxy-*N*-methylamphetamine (PMMA), *para*-methoxyethylamphetamine (PMEA), 4-fluoromethamphetamine (4-FMA), 4-chloroamphetamine (4-CA), 4-methylthioamphetamine (4-MTA), 2-fluoroamphetamine (2-FA), fenfluramine	137	Psychostimulatory, entactogenic, hallucinogenic (psychedelic)
Phenidate derivatives	Methylphenidate (MPH), ethylphenidate (EPH), propylphenidate (PPH), 4-fluoromethylphenidate (4F-MPH), 3,4-dichloromethylphenidate (3,4-DCMP), methylnaphthidate (HDMP-28)		Psychostimulatory
Aminorex analogues	Aminorex, 4-methylaminorex (4-MAR), 3,4-dimethylaminorex (3,4-DMAR), 4,4′-dimethylaminorex (4,4′-DMAR), 3′,4′-methylenedioxy-4-methylaminorex (MDMAR)		Psychostimulatory
Phenmetrazine derivatives	Phenmetrazine, 3-fluorophenmetrazine (3-FMP), 4-methylphenmetrazine (4-MPM)		Psychostimulatory
Thiophene designer drugs	Thiopropamine, methiopropamine (MPA)		Psychostimulatory
γ-Aminobutyric acid (GABA) analogues	γ-butyrolactone (GBL), γ-hydroxybutyric acid (GHB), γ-hydroxyvaleric acid (GHV), 4-amino-3-phenylbutyric acid (phenibut)		Sedative, hypnotic

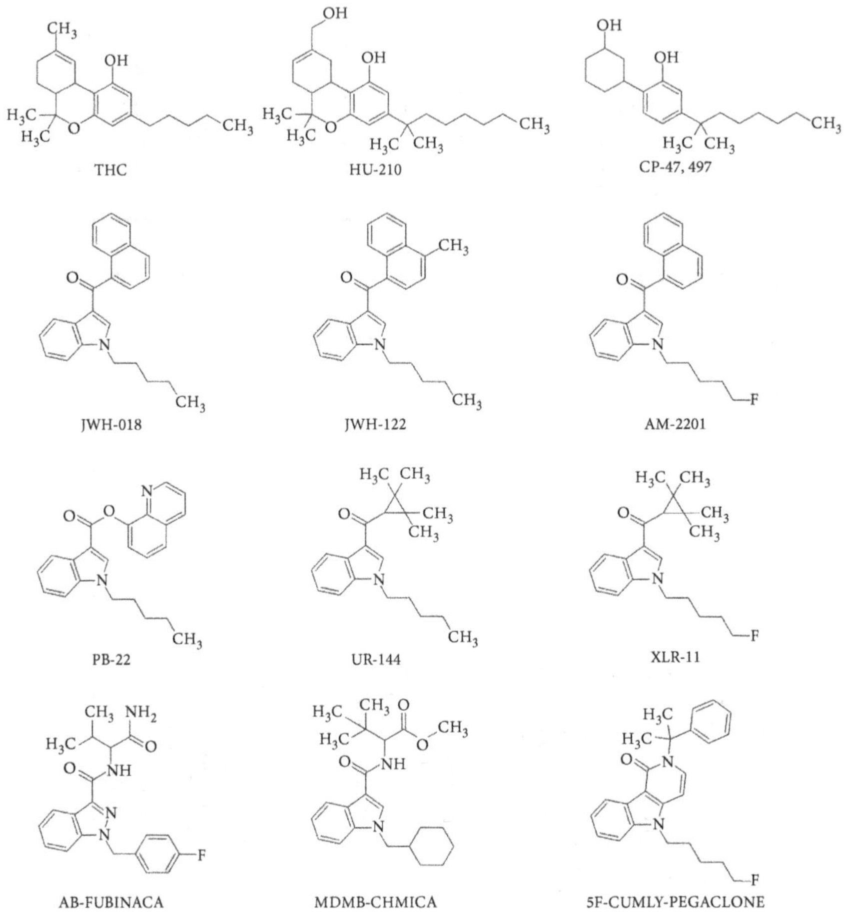

Figure 1.1. Exemplar structures of synthetic cannabinoids from different chemical groups.

hallucinations, delirium, and aggressive and violent behavior. Synthetic cannabinoids are likely to produce adverse effects atypical from those evoked by even high doses of cannabis/marijuana. Users may develop severe cardiovascular toxicity (including myocardial infarction), seizures, respiratory depression, pulmonary edema, rhabdomyolysis, nephrotoxicity, hyperemesis, and intracranial hemorrhages.[11] Adulterated cannabis may appear similar to unadulterated cannabis, and hence can be mis-sold as cannabis to unsuspecting consumers. An additional concern is a recently notified presence of synthetic cannabinoids in cannabis edibles in the form of sweets (jelly "gummies").[1]

Psychostimulants make up a broad group of diverse substances. The illicit drug market is dominated by synthetic cathinones. *Synthetic cathinones* (methcathinone and pyrovalerone derivatives) are analogues of a natural alkaloid cathinone occurring in fresh leaves of the khat (*Catha edulis*) shrub. Structurally they are β-keto analogues of amphetamine (Figure 1.2). Synthetic cathinones are available as white, yellowish, or brownish crystalline powder (hence they are commonly sold as "bath salts"), or as tablets or capsules that can be ingested or mixed up in the drink. By analogy to classical psychostimulants, snorting is a common way of using synthetic cathinones. Sometimes the powder is wrapped in a thin paper and swallowed (so-called "bombing") or dissolved and injected to achieve a fast onset of action. Synthetic cathinones potentiate brain signaling by elevating extracellular levels of monoamine neurotransmitters. They inhibit transporting proteins responsible for reuptake of dopamine, noradrenaline, and serotonin—DAT, NET, and SERT, respectively—into the presynaptic neuron. Some of them behave as substrates of transporter proteins and can induce release of these neurotransmitters. Desired effects of synthetic cathinones resemble those of

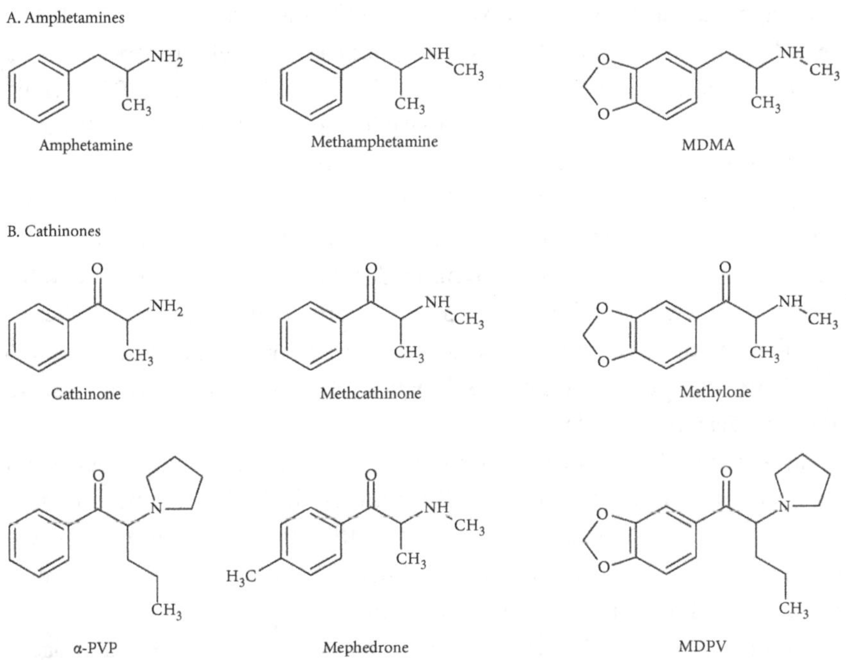

Figure 1.2. Exemplar structures of psychostimulants: (A) amphetamines and (B) synthetic cathinones.

cocaine, amphetamine, and MDMA (e.g., heightened alertness and awareness, increased energy and motivation, excitement, elevated mood, anorexia, and insomnia). Pyrovalerone derivatives, expressing higher affinity toward DAT over SERT, are potent psychostimulants endowed with a high abuse liability. On the other hand, methcathinones increase dopamine and serotonin neurotransmission equipotently or with a marked effect on serotonin and evoke mild empathogenic/entactogenic effects: openness in communication, empathy, sociability, talkativeness, and intensification of sensory perception.[6,12–14] It is worth mentioning that mephedrone is also used in a sexual context, particularly among groups of men who have sex with men, a phenomenon referred in the scientific literature as "chemsex" or "sexualized drug use."[15] Adverse effects related to use of synthetic cathinones mostly include agitation, aggression, restlessness, anxiety, hallucinations, psychosis, severe hyperthermia, tachycardia, hypertension, myocardial infarction, rhabdomyolysis, kidney injury, metabolic acidosis and respiratory alkalosis, and brain and pulmonary edema.[6,12–14] Recent reports indicate that the most popular synthetic cathinones included: 3-chloromethcathinone (3-CMC); 4-chloromethcathinone (4-CMC, clephedrone); 2-methylmethcathinone (2-MMC); 3-methylmethcathinone (3-MMC); 4-methylmethcathinone (4-MMC, mephedrone); *N*-ethylnorpentedrone; and α-pyrrolidinoizohexanophenone (α-PiHP). In 2022 and 2023 the EU Early Warning System noted an increase in reports of synthetic cathinones mis-sold as MDMA or used to adulterate MDMA.[1]

Other stimulants include piperazines, piperidines, pyrrolidines, aminoindanes, and new amphetamines. These compounds, when used at high doses, can also exhibit pronounced entactogenic or psychedelic-like effects by interacting with SERT and with serotonin receptors.[6,12] The less prevalent compounds with typically psychostimulatory properties include phenidate derivatives, aminorex analogues, phenmetrazine derivatives, and tiophene designer drugs.[6]

Hallucinogenic drugs can be divided into two groups: psychedelics and dissociatives. These substances are distinguished by high potency. Therefore, they are commonly used in the form of blotters (a minute, thin paper with absorbed drug, placed sublingually or buccally), rarely as tablets, powders, or liquids for intravenous use or vaporization.

Psychedelics, also known as classical/serotoninergic hallucinogens, create a chemically diverse group of indoleamines (lysergamides, simple tryptamines) and phenylalkylamines (phenylisopropylamines, 2C-X

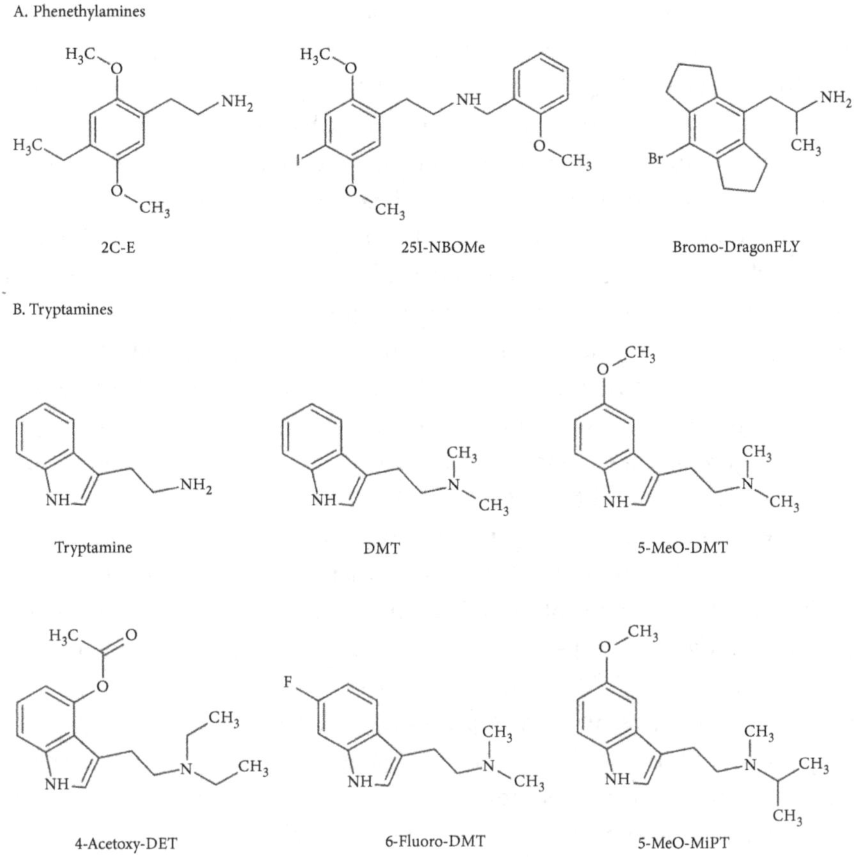

Figure 1.3. Exemplar structures of psychedelics: (A) phenethylamines and (B) tryptamines.

compounds and their analogues—NBOMes) (Figure 1.3). These substances are agonists of a variety of serotonin receptors with a high affinity for the 5-HT_{2A} receptor, stimulation of which is obligatory for psychedelic effects.[16] They elicit dreamlike alterations in consciousness (simple and complex visual imagery, distortion of perceiving the self and the surroundings), feelings, and thought processes.

Dissociative agents are mainly synthetic anesthetic drugs that disrupt capacity for information transmission in the brain. Consequently, a person experiences visual, auditory, and tactical hallucinations, depersonalization, derealization, disconnection from the body and environment, and seeing their own actions from a third-person perspective (out-of-body experience).

The main representatives of dissociatives include arylcyclohexamines and tryptamines. They act as *N*-methyl-D-aspartate (NMDA) receptor antagonists, decreasing the excitatory effects of glutamate and, as a result, the propagation of brain activity.[17] Although hallucinogens do not exert direct effects on brain dopamine circuits, which play a crucial role in the development of addiction, they may induce a vast array of adverse effects. Their distinctive negative effect is a hallucinogen-persisting perception disorder ("flashbacks"), for example, afterimages, perception of movement in peripheral visual fields, blurring of small patterns, flashes of various colors, enhanced color intensity, trailing and stroboscopic perception of moving objects, and halo effects. These episodes may persist for years.[18] Moreover, synthetic hallucinogens may evoke acute psychotic episodes, agitation (including aggressiveness), tachycardia, vasoconstriction, hypertension, and seizures eventually leading to death.[16,18]

In the group of *depressants*, synthetic opioids and designer, nonpharmaceutical benzodiazepines (DBZD) play a major role. *Synthetic opioids* are ligands for diverse types of opioid receptors in the brain and spinal cord, predominantly for the μ-type receptor that drives the main pharmacological effects of opioids. Activation of μ-opioid receptors produces euphoria, analgesia, respiratory depression, and development of addiction; δ-opioid receptors are responsible for analgesia and antidepressant effect, whereas κ-opioid receptors induce analgesia and hallucinogenic/dissociative effects, but also unpleasant mental states such as depression and dysphoria.[19] New synthetic opioids are establishing a strong position on the illegal drug market as stand-alone products, adulterants in heroin ("fake heroin"), or constituents of counterfeit prescription medications (e.g., hydromorphone, oxycodone, and falsified Xanax).[20] They have been one of the fastest-growing NPS subclasses in recent years, with 81 compounds detected in Europe between 2009 and 2023. Synthetic opioids comprise fentanyl and its analogues as well as compounds with different chemical structures, that is, diphenylethylpiperazines (e.g., MT-45 and its analogues), benzamide and 2-phenylacetamide opioids (so-called U-series), 2-benzylbenzimidazoles (nitazenes), and benzimidazolones (e.g., brorphine) (Figure 1.4 and Figure 1.5). The generic legislation outlawing fentanyl and its analogues contributed to a recent revival of research on opioids with distinct structures.[19,20] Of particular concern is the emergence of nitazenes, a class of synthetic opioids originally developed by pharmaceutical companies in the 1950s but never approved for therapeutic use (Figure 1.6).[1,3,21] Since 2019, the most frequently reported nitazenes include isotonitazene, metonitazene,

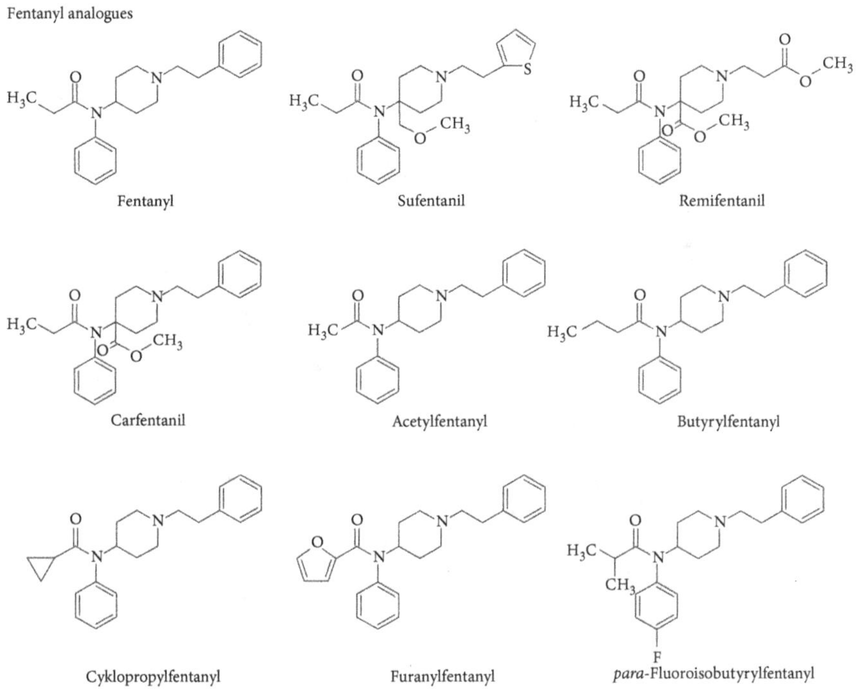

Figure 1.4. Exemplar structures of fentanyl analogues.

protonitazene, etonitazepyne, and etazene, all of which have since been placed under international control.[4] In the United Kingdom, nitazene abuse emerged in 2023 as an important cause of drug-overdose death, linked to 54 deaths over a 6-month period.[21] Illicit opioids are sold as powders, tablets, nasal sprays, and liquids. They generally display higher potency than morphine; for example, a potency of α-methylfentanyl is estimated to be 7000 times that of morphine, isotonitazene 500 times, etonitazene 1000 times, whereas carfentanil—even 10 000 times.[21,22] Therefore, they are mixed with heroin to increase its potency at a low cost and to falsify medicines—mostly prescription opioids and benzodiazepines.[8,19,20] Recently, alarming reports demonstrated an increase in popularity in the recreational street drug scene of xylazine, an animal sedative and analgesic drug, commonly mixed with heroin and illicit fentanyl ("tranq dope"), but sometimes also with new synthetic opioids that are not derivatives of fentanyl (e.g., protonitazene or metonitazene).[1,23,24] Considering the extremely high potency of synthetic opioids, their abuse poses a threat of central nervous system depression, respiratory arrest, pulmonary edema, coma, and even death.[8,19,20]

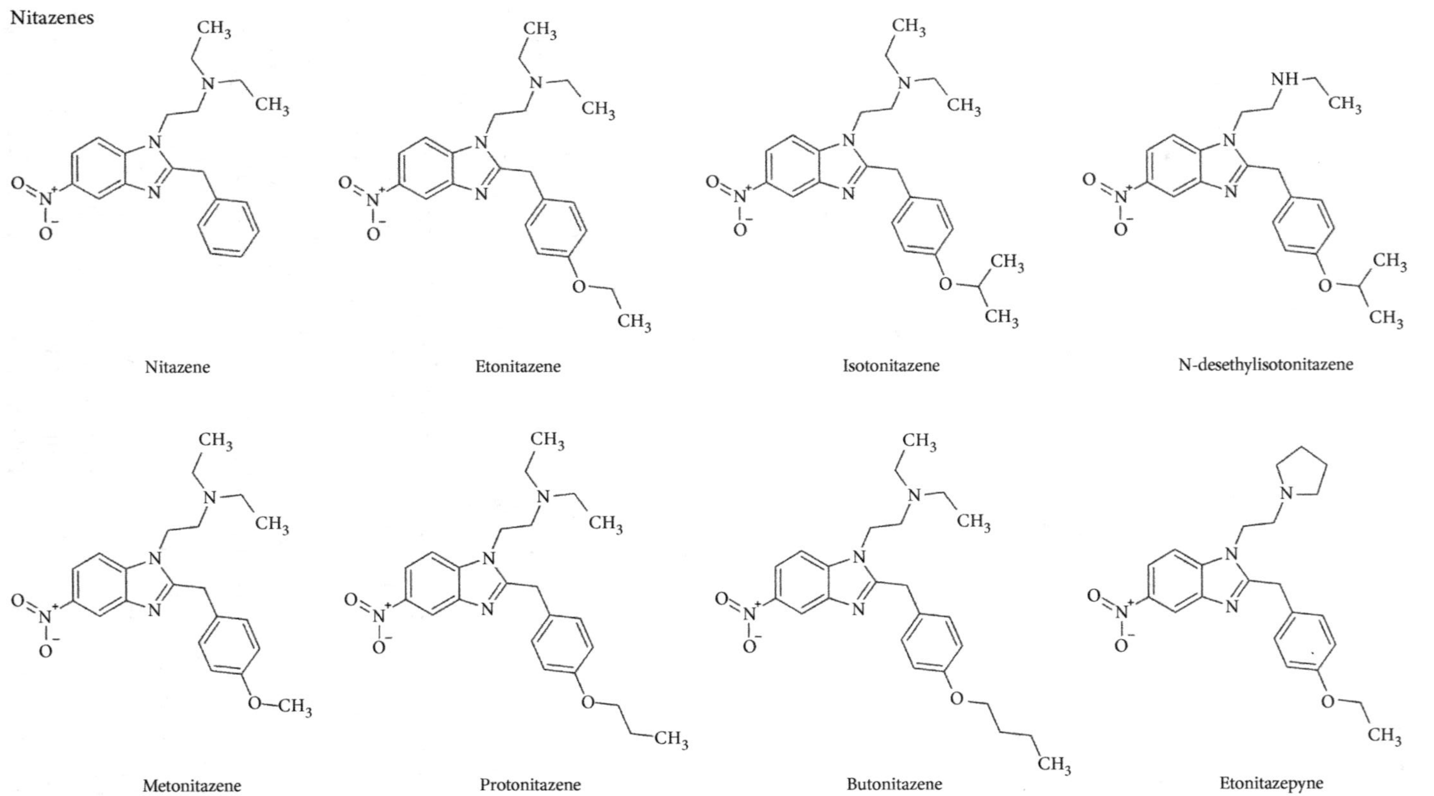

Figure 1.5. Exemplar structures of nitazenes.

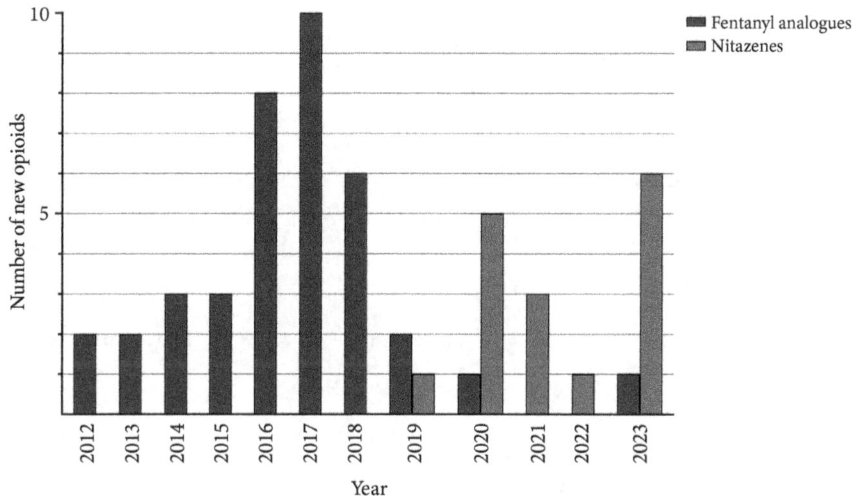

Figure 1.6. Number of fentanyl analogues and nitazenes monitored by EMCDDA.[1]

Designer benzodiazepines are positive allosteric modulators of γ-aminobutyric acid (GABA)-A receptors; they bind selectively to specific sites located on α subunits of these receptors, enhancing effects mediated by an endogenous inhibitory neurotransmitter GABA (i.e., anxiolytic, sedative, hypnotic, anterograde amnesic, anticonvulsant, and myorelaxant). Chemically DBZD belong to 1,4-benzodiazepines (a typical structure of classical BZD), triazolo- and thienotriazolobenzodiazepines (Figure 1.7). The DBZD group of NPS comprises pharmacological drug candidates that have never earned approval for medical use (e.g., clonazolam, diclazepam, flubromazepam, meclozepam, and pyrazolam) or those legally prescribed in a few countries (e.g., phenazepam and etizolam). Some compounds derive from registered drugs; for example, diclazepam and 4′-chlorodiazepam are chlorine-substituted derivatives of diazepam. Others are active metabolites of prescription drugs that emerge as NPS; for example, fonazepam (desmethylflunitrazepam) and nifoxipam (3-hydroxydesmethylflunitrazepam) are active metabolites of flunitrazepam (Rohypnol)—a very potent hypnotic benzodiazepine, used rarely as a prescription drug but more frequently as a so-called "rape drug." DBZD are offered at low prices under their own names in the form of tablets, pills, capsules, pellets, powders, blotters, and liquids. Some are pressed into counterfeit tablets strikingly imitating existing medicines, like alprazolam

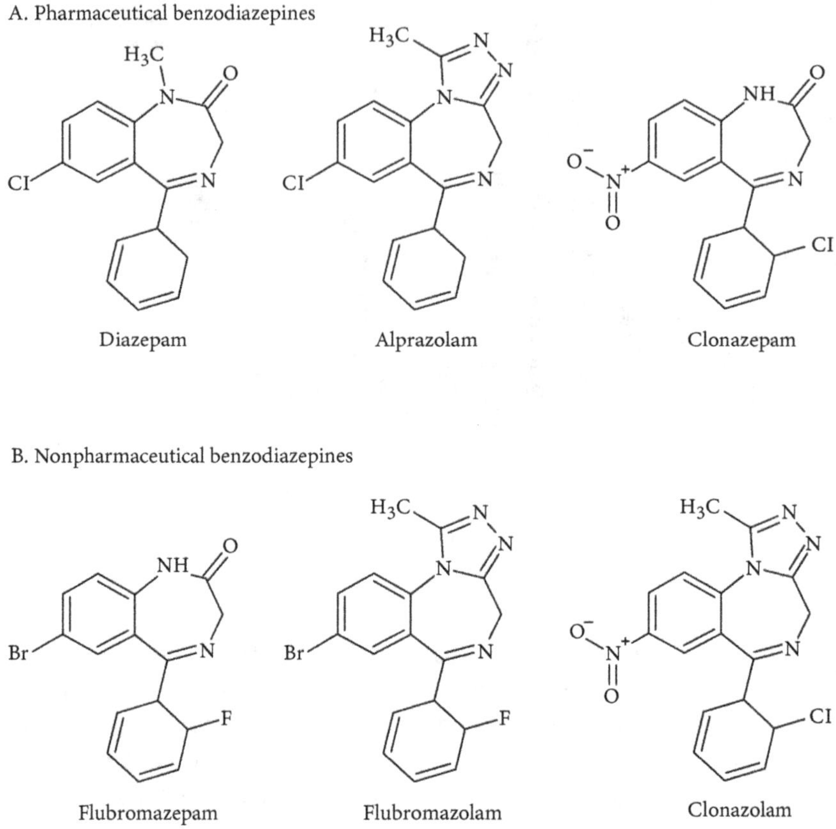

Figure 1.7. Exemplar structures of benzodiazepines: (A) pharmaceutical benzodiazepines and (B) nonpharmaceutical benzodiazepines.

(Xanax) and diazepam (Relanium). The range of elimination phase after oral intake varies significantly among different DBZD: from short-acting drugs such as etizolam with a half-life about 3 hours, to long-acting drugs (e.g., phenazepam and flubromazepam) with a half-life of 103 hours and 106 hours, respectively. The delayed onset of action poses a risk of overdose/intoxication after re-dosing drugs when an initial dose has not been experienced. Additionally, after repeated use the long-acting DBZD are likely to accumulate in tissues. Although isolated use of DBZD is rarely fatal, they may induce delirium, auditory and visual hallucinations, deep sleep, and coma at high doses.[25]

An alternative group of sedatives that became available as designer drugs are analogues of natural neurotransmitter GABA, for example, γ-hydroxybutyric acid (GHB) and γ-butyrolactone (GBL), which induce euphoria and relaxation, reduce social anxiety, and increase sexual drive, but their safety margin is significantly narrower than those of DBZD as they can act directly on GABA receptors.[6]

1.4. NPS of Natural Origin

A wide range of naturally derived substances have been abused for millennia since humans serendipitously discovered psychoactive properties of compounds present in plants, fungi, or even animals. To the globally used classical drugs that are plant-derived belong opium (dried juice from unripe poppy capsules of *Papaver somniferum*), cocaine in the leaves of *Erythroxylon coca*, and cannabis (*Cannabis sativa*) with its phytochemical products—marijuana and hashish containing significant amounts of Δ^9-THC.[26] The majority of plants containing psychoactive substances grow in South America, Asia, and Africa, and for a long time their use has been restricted to the area of a natural occurrence. Since they allow users to experience an altered state of mind and perception by evoking relaxing, sedative, hypnotic, hallucinogenic, and stimulating/analeptic effects, they have been commonly used in religious rituals, cultural events, or in traditional medicine as pain relievers.[27] Although synthetic NPS have dominated the market of recreational drugs, NPS of natural origin have grown in importance and have spread across the world through online vendors. In addition, natural products also give rise to new, broad classes of NPS, such as synthetic cannabinoids and synthetic cathinones. The main plant-derived NPS and their pharmacological properties are presented in Table 1.2.

1.5. NPS Products

On the drug market, products containing NPS are usually offered under colloquial terms like "designer drugs," "legal highs," "research chemicals," "party pills," "herbal highs," "herbal mixtures," "bath salts," "plant food," "fertilizers," "incenses," "Halloween candies," "pound cleaners," "air fresheners," "potpourri," and so on, to sell them freely and encourage their further spread.[2,28,29] Moreover, they are often intentionally mislabeled with the disclaimer "not for human consumption" or "for scientific research only" to further surpass

Table 1.2 Psychoactive Substances of Natural Origins

Species/ Genus	Common Name(s)	Region of Origin	Plant/Fungi Part	Main Psychoactive Compound(s)	Mechanism of action	Activity profile
Arecha catechu	Betel quid	Asia (Sri Lanka, Malaysia)	Areca nut (fruit)	Arecoline	GABA competitive inhibitor; non-selective nicotinic and muscarinic receptor antagonist	Psychostimulatory, relaxing, aphrodisiac
Argyreia nervosa	Adhoguda, vidhara, elephant creeper, *Rivea corymbosa*, Hawaiian baby woodrose, morning glory, *Ipomoea violacea*	India	Seeds	Isoergine, lysergamide (LSA)	5-HT_{2A} receptor agonists	Psychedelic
Banister-eriopsis caapi, Psychotria viridins	Ayahuasca caapi, daime, hoasca, yage, natema	South America (Amazon)	Decoction of *B. caapi* shavings from the stem and *P. viridis* leaves	*N,N*-dimethyltryptamine (DMT) + β-carbolinic alkaloids:harmine,harmaline, tetrahydroharmine (THH)	$5\text{-HT}_{1A/2A/2C}$ receptor agonist (DMT), MAO-A inhibitors (β-carbolines), serotonin reuptake inhibitor (THH)	Hallucinogenic
Catha edulis	Khat, qat, kafta	Horn of Africa, Arabian peninsula	Fresh leaves	S-(−)-cathinone, cathine ([S,S-(+)-norpseudoephedrine]), phenylpropanolamine	Inhibiting reuptake and/or increasing release of DA, NA, 5-HT	Amphetamine-like (psychostimulatory, anorectic)
Datura stramonium	Jimson weed	Central America, early spread to Europe, Asia, and Africa	Dried leaves, flowers, seeds	Scopolamine, atropine	Muscarinic receptors antagonists	Hallucinogenic

Lophophora williamsii	Peyote	Northern Mexico, United States	Flesh of the fresh cactus	Mescaline	5-$HT_{1A/2A/2C}$ receptor agonist	Hallucinogenic
Mandragora officinarium	Mandrake	Eastern Mediterranean	Seeds, roots, leaves, fruits	Hyoscyamine, atropine, scopolamine	Muscarinic receptors antagonists	Hallucinogenic
Mitragyna speciosa	Kratom	Asia (Cambodia, Thailand, Indonesia, Malaysia, and Myanmar), Papua New Guinea	Fresh or dried leaves	Mitragynine, 7-hydroxymitragynine, corinantheidine, speciogினine, paynantheine	μ-opioid receptor partial agonist, δ-opioid receptor antagonist (mitragynine)	Opioid-like (analgesic, euphoric)
Piper methysticum	Kava	Pacific region	Roots, stems	Kavalactones (kavain, yangonin, desmethoxyiangonin, 7,8-dihydrokavain, methysticin, 7,8-dihydromethysticin)	MAO-B inhibitors, NA and DA reuptake inhibitors, allosteric modulation of $GABA_A$ receptors' function	Anxiolytic, analgesic, hypnotic
Psilocybe	Magic mushrooms	Mexico	Whole mushrooms, capsules, tea of dried mushrooms	Psylocibin psylocin	5-$HT_{1A/2A}$ receptors agonist, Glutamate release (agonist of NMDA receptors)	Hallucinogenic
Salvia divinorum	Hierba di Maria	Mexico (Oaxaca region)	Fresh or dried leaves	Salvinorin A	Selective agonist of κ-opioid receptor	Hallucinogenic
Tabernanthe iboga		Central and West Africa	Dry root bark	Ibogaine	σ2 receptor agonist, nicotinic α3β4 acetylcholine receptor antagonist, NMDA receptor antagonist	Psychostimulatory, hallucinogenic

DA: dopamine; GABA: γ-aminobutyric acid; 5-HT: serotonin; MAO: monoamine oxidase; NA: noradrenaline; NMDA: N-methyl-D-aspartate the legislation and escape from responsibility in cases of serious/fatal intoxication of consumers.[2] Some NPS are even advertised as a safer version of well-known drugs of abuse; for example, methoxetamine, a potent dissociative, is being offered as a "bladder-friendly" alternative to ketamine.[7]

NPS are being sold in a variety of formulations; packages containing them are colorful and eye-catching, as they are typically directed to adolescents and young adults. Brand names of NPS products refer not only to movies, comics, animals, and landscape/space, but also directly to expected psychotropic effects (e.g., "Tripstasy," "Mr. Happy," "45 Minutes Psychosis," "Bliss," "Trip," "Blurberrys").[29,30] Some names even relate to the controlled drugs: "Coco Power," "Crack Inside," "EXTC," "Xtacy."[13] The same street name stands for various NPS in different countries or at different times, making it difficult to track the popularity of particular substances. Thus, within different series of the same product, various chemical substances can be identified. It should be emphasized that NPS are rapidly rebranded. For instance, JWH-018, a popular synthetic cannabinoid in the early 2000s, was sold under several names, including "Kryptonite," "Black Widow," "King Cobra," "K2," "Moon Rocks," "Dr. Feel Good," "Mr. Nice Guy," among others.[27]

As the NPS products might lack labeling, or their label claim may not correspond to the actual active compound(s), consumers can never be sure what exactly they take and at what dose. Furthermore, "legal highs" may contain a single psychoactive ingredient, but more often they constitute a drug mixture with a wide range of impurities, adulterants, or diluents. Common adulterants used to mimic or antagonize the effects of the main drug are: topical anesthetics (benzocaine, lidocaine, procaine), caffeine, levamisole, and paracetamol, while inactive diluents increasing the bulk of the products include lactose, microcrystalline cellulose, and talc.[29] NPS are often used as adulterants, thus users may be unaware that they are using NPS, meaning that they cannot report their use in a survey. Furthermore, it is not uncommon for users to be unable to categorize the substance(s) they have used within the given categories.[9]

1.6. Current Trends

As a "cat and mouse game" regarding legislation policy continued, the number of available NPS exerting various psychopharmacological effects rose dramatically. After reaching its peak in 2014 with 101 NPS detected in Europe for the first time, the number of emerging drugs has declined. Between 2017 and 2021 the number of newly detected substances oscillated around 50 per year. According to the latest EMCDDA drug report, the number of newly identified NPS in Europe fell to 41 in 2022, whereas in 2023 only 26 new compounds were notified. These changes may be explained by an introduction of more restrictive regulations, including so-called "blanket bans" and generic/analogue legislations in some countries. Nevertheless, it is estimated that around 400 previously reported NPS are detected on the European market each year.[1] In 2022 there were 566 NPS available on the global market, slightly less than in the previous year. Although the pace of new substances being introduced to the market may be slowing, the overall number of substances is growing incessantly as new substances are continuously added to the list (Figure 1.8 and Figure 1.9).[1,3] At the end of 2023, the EMCDDA was monitoring around 950 NPS, while the global number of NPS reported to the UNODC was 1,240.[1,3] At present the highest number of NPS refers to synthetic cannabinoids; though in terms of effect groups, the highest number concerns synthetic stimulants, mostly cathinones and, to a lesser extent, phenethylamines. Among plant-based NPS, the most frequently seized products are khat and kratom. Overall, the consumption of

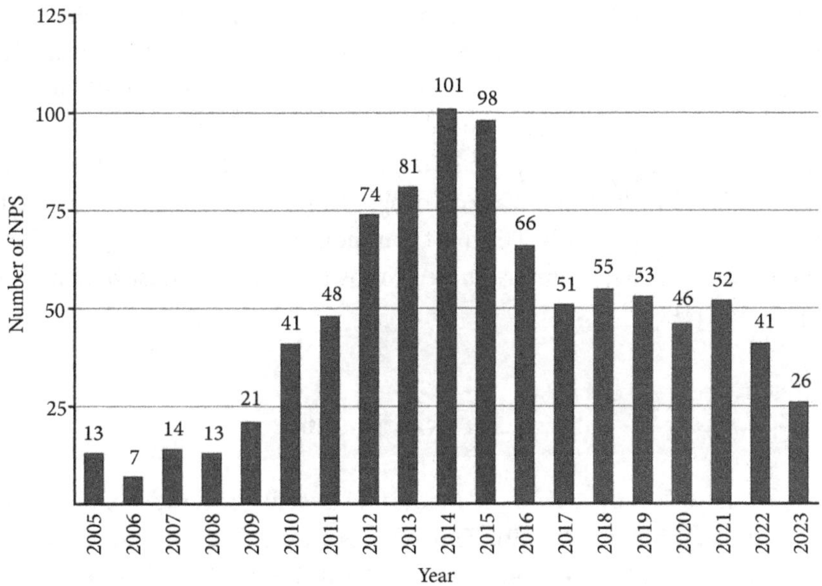

Figure 1.8. Number of NPS notified for the first time to the European Monitoring Centre for Drugs and Drugs Addiction each year during 2005–2023.[1]

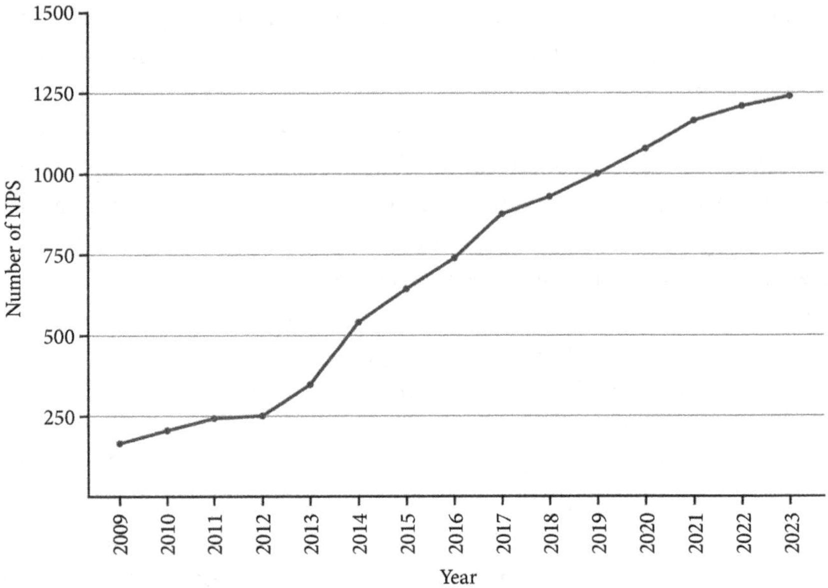

Figure 1.9. Total number of NPS monitored by United Nations Office on Drugs and Crime, 2009–2023.[3]

NPS is lower than that of classical drugs of abuse. However, despite a certain tendency of declining use of NPS in Europe and North America, NPS trafficking further expands its geographical reach to low- and middle-income countries in Eastern Europe, Central Asia, and Africa, where the control systems are weaker.[3] Currently, we also observe a worldwide trend of selling products laced with NPS as classical drugs of abuse or well-established medicine to unsuspecting users. The most common adulterants are new synthetic opioids and DBZD; therefore these groups are also the most dynamically developing NPS.[1,3]

Acknowledgments

This work was supported by the Medical University of Lodz, Poland (grant 503/3-011-01/503-31-002-19). The authors would like to thank Professor Piotr Adamowicz from the Institute of Forensic Research in Cracow, Poland, for the figures of chemical structures of major NPS representatives.

References

1. EMCDDA. European Drug Report 2024. Trends and developments: New psychoactive substances—the current situation in Europe. 2024. https://www.euda.europa.eu/publications/european-drug-report/2024/new-psychoactive- substances_en. Accessed July 8, 2024.
2. UNODC. World Drug Report 2013. 2013. https://www.unodc.org/unodc/secured/wdr/wdr2013/World_Drug_Report_2013.pdf. Accessed June 24, 2022.
3. UNODC. World Drug Report 2024. 2024a. https://www.unodc.org/unodc/en/data-and-analysis/wdr2024-drug-market-trends. Accessed July 8, 2024.
4. UNODC. UNODC EWA: Nitazenes—a new group of synthetic opioids emerges. 2024b. https://www.unodc.org/LSS/Announcement/Details/cbec8f4c-73aa-49ee-9e2b-75620af8a910. Accessed July 13, 2024.
5. Council of the European Union. Council Decision 2005/387/JHA of 10 May 2005 on the information exchange, risk-assessment and control of new psychoactive substances. *Official J Eur Union.* 2005;L127:32–37.
6. Luethi D, Liechti ME. Designer drugs: Mechanism of action and adverse effects. *Arch Toxicol.* 2020;94(4):1085–1133. https://doi.org/10.1007/s00204-020-02693-7. Erratum in: *Arch Toxicol.* 2022;96(5):1489. https://doi.org/10.1007/s00204-022-03244-y
7. EMCDDA. Europol 2013 Annual Report of the implementation of Council Decision 2005/387/JHA. 2013. https://www.emcdda.europa.eu/attachements.cfm/att_229598_EN_TDAN14001ENN.pdf. Accessed June 24, 2022.
8. Zawilska JB. An expanding world of novel psychoactive substances: Opioids. *Front Psychiatry.* 2017;8:110. https://doi.org/10.3389/fpsyt.2017.00110.
9. UNODC. World Drug Report 2022. Booklet 4: Drug market trends. Cocaine, amphetamine-type stimulants, new psychoactive substances. 2022. https://www.unodc.org/res/wdr2022/MS/WDR22_Booklet_4.pdf. Accessed July 10, 2022.
10. Shafi A, Berry AJ, Sumnall H, Wood DM, Tracy DK. New psychoactive substances: A review and updates. *Ther Adv Psychopharmacol.* 2020;10:1–21. https://doi.org/10.1177/2045125320967197.
11. Zawilska JB, Kuczyńska K, Bratzu J, Fattore L. Neurotoxicity of exogenous cannabinoids. In: Kostrzewa RM, ed. *Handbook of Neurotoxicity.* Springer; 2022:1323–1353. https://doi.org/10.1007/978-3-031-15080-7_206.
12. Milliano C, Serpelloni G, Rimondo C, Mereu M, Marti M, De Luca MA. Neuropharmacology of new psychoactive substances (NPS): Focus on the rewarding and reinforcing properties of cannabimimetics and amphetamine-like stimulants. *Front Neurosci.* 2016;10:153. https://doi.org/10.3389/fnins.2016.00153.
13. Zawilska JB, Wojcieszak J. Designer cathinones: An emerging class of novel recreational drugs. *Forensic Sci Int.* 2013;231(1–3):42–53. https://doi.org/10.1016/j.forsciint.2013.04.015.
14. Zawilska JB, Wojcieszak J. α-Pyrrolidinophenones: A new wave of designer cathinones. *Forensic Toxicol.* 2017;35(2):201–216. https://doi.org/10.1007/s11419-016-0353-6.
15. Coronado-Muñoz M, García-Cabrera E, Quintero-Flórez A, Román E, Vilches-Arenas Á. Sexualized drug use and chemsex among men who have sex with men in Europe: A systematic review and meta-analysis. *J Clin Med.* 2024;13(6):1812. https://doi.org/10.3390/jcm13061812.
16. Zawilska JB, Kacela M, Adamowicz P. NBOMes: Highly potent and toxic alternatives of LSD. *Front Neurosci.* 2020;14:78. https://doi.org/10.3389/fnins.2020.00078.
17. Sanz C, Zamberlan F, Erowid E, Erowid F, Tagliazucchi E. The experience elicited by hallucinogens presents the highest similarity to dreaming within a large database of psychoactive substance reports. *Front Neurosci.* 2018;12:7. https://doi.org/10.3389/fnins.2018.00007. Erratum in: *Front Neurosci.* 2018;12:229. https://doi.org/10.3389/fnins.2018.00229.

18. Nicols DE. Psychedelics. *Pharmacol Rev.* 2016;68(2):264–355. https://doi.org/10.1124/pr.115.011478. Erratum in: *Pharmacol Rev.* 2016;68(2):356. doi:10.1124/pr.114.011478err.
19. Hasegawa K, Minakata K, Suzuki M, Osamu S. Non-fentanyl-derived synthetic opioids emerging during recent years. *Forensic Toxicol.* 2022;40(2):234–243. https://doi.org/10.1007/s11419-022-00624-y.
20. Zawilska JB, Adamowicz P, Kurpeta M, Wojcieszak J. Non-fentanyl new synthetic opioids: An update. *Forensic Sci Int.* 2023;349:111775. https://doi.org/10.1016/j.forsciint.2023.111775.
21. Holland A, Copeland CS, Shorter GW, et al. Nitazenes-heralding a second wave for the UK drug-related death crisis? *Lancet Public Health.* 2024;9(2):e71–e72. https://doi.org/10.1016/S2468-2667(24)00001-X.
22. Lovrecic B, Lovrecic M, Gabrovec B, et al. Non-medical use of novel synthetic opioids: A new challenge to public health. *Int J Environ Res Public Health.* 2019;16(2):177. https://doi.org/10.3390/ijerph16020177.
23. EMCDDA. European Drug Report 2023. Trends and developments: New psychoactive substances—the current situation in Europe. 2023. https://www.euda.europa.eu/publications/european-drug-report/2023/new-psychoactive-substances_en. Accessed July 8, 2024.
24. Hoffman GR, Giduturi C, Cordaro NJ, et al. Classics in Chemical Neuroscience: Xylazine. *ACS Chem Neurosci.* 2024;15(11):2091–2098. https://doi.org/10.1021/acschemneuro.4c00172.
25. Zawilska JB, Wojcieszak J. An expanding world of new psychoactive substances: Designer benzodiazepines. *Neurotoxicology.* 2019;73:8–16. https://doi.org/10.1016/j.neuro.2019.02.015.
26. Feng L-Y, Battulga A, Han E, Chung H, Li J-H. New psychoactive substances of natural origin: A brief review. *J Food Drug Anal.* 2017;25(3):461–471. https://doi.org/10.1016/j.jfda.2017.04.001.
27. Gonçalves J, Luís Â, Gallardo E, Duarte AP. Psychoactive substances of natural origin: Toxicological aspects, therapeutic properties and analysis in biological samples. *Molecules.* 2021;26(5):1397. https://doi.org/10.3390/molecules26051397.
28. Zawilska JB. Legal highs—An emerging epidemic of novel psychoactive substances. *Int Rev Neurobiol.* 2015;120:273–300. https://doi.org/10.1016/bs.irn.2015.02.009.
29. Corazza O, Valeriani G, Bersani FS, et al. "Spice," "kryptonite," "black mamba": An overview of brand names and marketing strategies of novel psychoactive substances on the web. *J Psychoact Drugs.* 2014;46(4):287–294. https://doi.org/10.1080/02791072.2014.944291.
30. Assi S, Guirguis A, Halsey S, Fergus S, Stair JL. Analysis of "legal high" substances and common adulterants using handheld spectroscopic technique. *Anal Methods.* 2015;7(2):736–746. https://doi.org/10.1039/c4ay02169j.

2

The Pandemic of NPS in Society

An Overview of the Social Context

Elisabeth Prevete, Giuseppe Bersani, and Ornella Corazza

2.1. Background of an Ever-Evolving Phenomenon

New psychoactive substances (NPS), also known as "synthetic or designer drugs," are "substances of abuse, either in a pure form or a preparation, that are not controlled by the 1961 Single Convention on Narcotic Drugs or the 1971 Convention on Psychotropic Substances, but which may pose a public health threat,"[1(n.p.)] and which include a wide range of products.

Although NPS vary in terms of chemical and pharmacodynamic profile, they can be grouped according to their effects in the following categories[2,3] (Figure 2.1): stimulants (synthetic cathinones [SCs], piperazines, tryptamines, 2C phenylethylamines); synthetic hallucinogens (dissociative and hallucinogenic NPS); synthetic cannabinoid receptor agonists (SCRA, the most used NPS with SCs);[4,5] synthetic depressants (opioids and sedatives/hypnotics); plant-based substances (e.g., ayahuasca, khat, kratom, salvia divinorum); and others, such as products used as image- and performance-enhancing drugs (IPEDs), which represent the new challenge of this novel drug scene.

Since the appearance of the first NPS ("Spice" products) over a decade ago,[6] the drugs scenario has constantly evolved with the emergence of a wide range of new compounds leading to an unprecedented "growing worldwide epidemic."[7,8(n.p.)]

Data on NPS use derive mainly from case series and case reports, while findings from epidemiological investigations across the general population remain scarce. So far over 850 illicit substances have been officially identified in 119 countries and territories by the United Nations Office on Drugs and Crime (UNODC)'s Global SMART (Synthetics Monitoring: Analyses, Reporting and Trends) Programme[9] and the European Monitoring Centre for Drugs and Drug Addiction (EMCDDA)'s Early Warning Systems (EWS).[10]

In this scenario, NPS are often marketed with different brand names as "research chemicals," "legal highs," or "not for human consumption" and are advertised, in pure form or mixed with other substances, as a "legal and cheaper alternative" to classical controlled substances (e.g., LSD, cannabis),[3,11] sometimes found as adulterants in supplements and IPEDs, which are typically sold as "natural" and "safer" alternatives to pharmaceutical compounds.

Such products are easily available on the internet and elsewhere, with social media (e.g., Facebook, X, Instagram) and mobile communication applications (apps) playing an increasing role on their diffusion. In a globalized society, such new tools of communication have facilitated the NPS sales, supply, and delivery[12–14] in ways that cannot be compared to the past, creating new forms of concerns in terms of public health and international legislative controls.

Attention has also been given to the availability of NPS on the "darknet" ("dark web"). Such illicit drug markets are accessible only with special software operating with anonymity and crypto currencies having The Onion

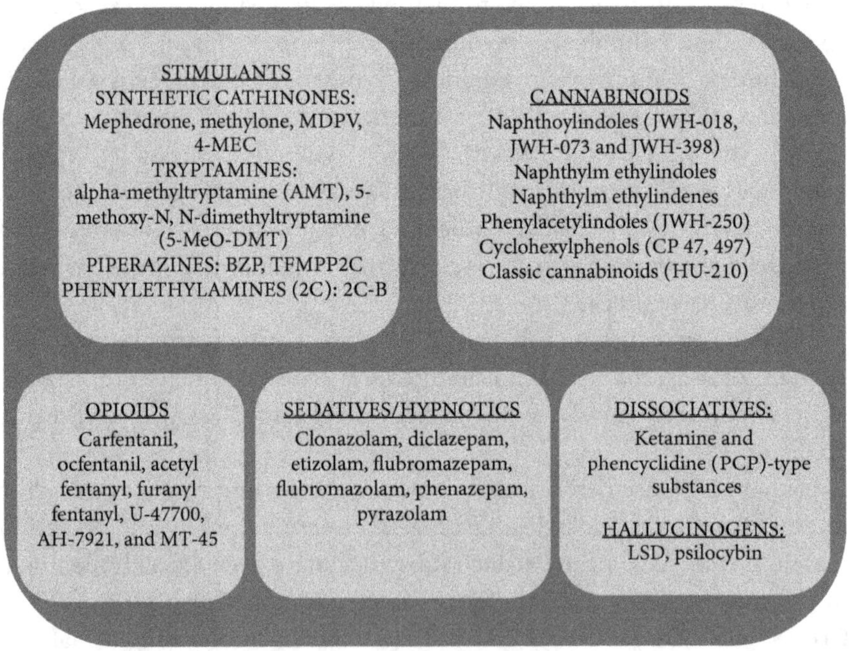

Figure 2.1. Main NPS groups.

Router (TOR) as host,[13,14] creating new business for large organized crime groups (OCG).[13] Since their first appearance in 2010, more than 100 global darknet markets have been identified,[10] with an estimated profit of EUR 800,000 per day in the period from July 2017 to August 2018.[15]

2.2. NPS User Profile: Between the Old and the New Trends

We currently know that NPS use is mostly diffuse among young adults, mainly males,[4,16–18] and adolescents, and that NPS are often taken in association with the use of other substances (e.g., cannabis, alcohol).[19] A typical NPS user is often a polydrug user who has used drugs before.[20,21] Stronger sensation seeking and impulsivity traits have also been identified among such a cohort in comparison to other illicit- and non-drug users.[22]

The motivations for drug use also have dramatically changed over the past decades (Figure 2.2), leading to the increased consumption of image- and performance-enhancing drugs (IPEDs) to boost physical and cognitive performance,[23,24] which were once limited to competitive sport environments.[25]

Among NPS users we find not only the typical recreational users or "psychonauts,"[26] but also college students and professionals;[24] gym-goers;[27] club-goers;[28] military personnel, drivers, and pilots;[24] prisoners;[23] homeless persons;[29] farmers (to combat fatigue);[30] subjects suffering from chronic pain (who claim to seek the benefits of some plant-based medicines, such as kratom);[31] and psychiatric patients (who are inclined to use NPS to self-medicate their conditions).[32]

2.3. NPS Use: Motivations and Patterns in the Globalized Social Context

The main underlying motivations for NPS use, regardless of their category, include pragmatic (practical/economical) reasons, such as (1) low price; (2) attractive packaging; (3) legal status; (4) home production and easy accessibility on the internet; (5) presumed purity of the products; and (6) non-detectability in urine and blood sample tests used as screening tools.[11,33,34]

Other motives for NPS use include: (1) curiosity, recreational purposes, and enhancing creativity;[35,36] (2) pleasure, enjoyment (e.g., "enjoying

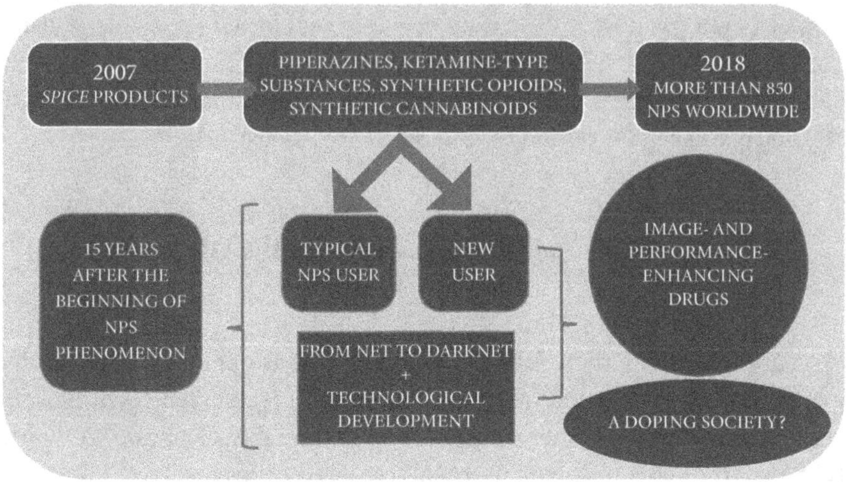

Figure 2.2. Evolution of the NPS scenario.

intoxication" or "having a good time"), and social enhancement;[11,37] (3) self-assertion in achieving personal goals;[24] (4) self-exploration (e.g., psychonauts)[26] and coping strategy, especially during the COVID-19 pandemic, with restrictions and quarantine having potentially contributed to an increase in addictive behaviors;[38,39] and dark web use among individuals without previous experience.

Despite this general background, motivations for NPS use might vary between NPS groups and user groups' characteristics. The next sections will discuss each of these groups while taking into account the wider social context.

2.3.1. Synthetic Stimulants

According to Graddy, Buresh, and Rastegar,[2] synthetic stimulants are considered those designer drugs resembling psychoactive effects of traditional stimulant drugs (e.g., MDMA, amphetamines, cocaine) and include synthetic cathinones and other compounds which, according to other authors,[3] belong to the group of synthetic hallucinogens, such as synthetic piperazines, tryptamines, and 2C phenylethylamines (2C).

Synthetic cathinones (SCs), such as 4-methylmethcathinone (mephedrone, 4-MMC), 3,4-methylenedioxy-N-methylcathinone (methylone), 3,4-methylenedioxypyrovalerone (MDPV), 4-methyl-N-ethylcathinone (4-MEC), 4-fluoromethcathinone (flephedrone,

4-FMC), 3-fluoromethcathinone (3-FMC), and α-PVP (α-pyrrolidinopentiophenone), are known in the social context by different brand names (e.g., Bath Salts, Plant Food, Meow-Meow, m-CAT, Bubbles, Bounce, Ivory Wave, Vanilla Sky, Energy-1).[2,3]

By resembling the effect of khat, a psychoactive substance contained in the *Catha edulis* plant, SCs act on monoamine (dopamine [DA], serotonine [5HT], and noradrenaline [NE]) transporters[40] and are available in several formulations (e.g., powder, capsules, crystals, tablets, pills, and water solutions). They can be consumed via a range of routes, for example, oral intake (the most commonly used route), nasal insufflation, inhalation, smoking, injection, or rectally, often in combination with other substances (e.g., alcohol, cocaine, ecstasy, cannabis).[2,3,40]

The social context typical of SC use is represented by exchange programs involving injecting drug users (IDU)[41] and recreational settings (e.g., nightclubs, home party, bar) as well, sometimes including the so-called "mephedrone sessions" (repeated consumption of SCs in a short time) or the *slam practice*, which refers to intravenous administration of psychoactive substances to enhance both pleasure and sexual performance during "chem-sex" parties,[40] especially among men having sex with men (MSM). Main reported reasons of SC use include practical or economical aspects (as for all NPS),[40] curiosity, replacement of other drugs (e.g., heroin or other stimulants,[42] and, as claimed by users, self-treating of some conditions (e.g., anxiety, depression, and attention deficit hyperactivity disorder [ADHD]).

Piperazine derivatives include both benzylpiperazine and phenylpiperazine derivatives, such as N-benzylpiperazine (BZP), 1-(3,4-methylenedioxybenzyl)piperazine (MDBP), 1-(4-fluorobenzyl)piperazine (pFBP), 1,4-dibenzylpiperazine (DBZP), 1-(3-trifluoro-methylphenyl) piperazine (TFMPP), 1-(3-chlorophenyl)piperazine (mCPP), 1-(4-parafluoro-phenyl)piperazine (pFPP), and 1-(4-methoxyphenyl)piperazine (MeOPP).[2,43] These designer drugs are known in the social context by the following brand names: Frenzy, Legal X, Legal E, Bliss, A2, Benny Bear, Flying Angel, Rapture, Charge, Herbal Ecstasy, Twisted, Jax, Nemesis, Red Eye Frog. By exerting amphetamine-like effects and acting on monoamine transporters, they are mainly used as alternatives to 3,4-methylenedioxymethamphetamine (MDMA).[2,43] Available in the form of powder, injection, tablets, party pills, solutions, or sometimes as adulterants (e.g., with caffeine or herbal extracts), piperazines derivatives are often combined with other club drugs (e.g., ecstasy, amphetamine, ketamine) and mainly are consumed per oral intake[2,43] in recreational settings (e.g., electronic dance clubs, raves, pubs, bars).[2,43] Among the main reasons behind their use, pragmatic features, enjoying psychoactive/hallucinogenic effects, and the need to improve image and mental or body performance[43,44] have been reported.

Synthetic tryptamines, such as alpha-methyltryptamine (AMT), N,N-dimethyltryptamine (DMT), N,N-diallyl-5-methoxytryptamine (5-MeO-DALT), 5-methoxy-N,N-dimethyltryptamine (5-MeO-DMT), and 5-methoxy-N, N-diisopropyltryptamine (5-MeO-DIPT), are commonly diffuse in the social context with the Foxy or Plant Food brand names.[2,3] Such synthetic compounds act on 5HT2A receptors. By resembling the effect of psychoactive substances in ayahuasca and psilocybin, they exert psychedelic (e.g., ability to induce ASC, modification of self-perception, mood, thoughts) and stimulant effects.[2,3,45] Tryptamines are sold as tablets, powders, pills, and blotter paper, with users consuming them per oral intake, or even through other routes (e.g., nasal insufflation, inhalation, smoking, injection), often in combination with other substances (e.g., monoamine oxidase inhibitors).[2,3,45] Tryptamine use is typical of recreational contexts, such as raves or nightclubs, where users choose such drugs for practical motivations (e.g., easily available over the internet) and the desire to experience psychedelic sensations (e.g., ego loss, novel insights, increased intensity of music and colors).[45,46]

Two-carbon (2C) phenethylamines include a broad class of substances such as 2,5-dimethoxy-4-bromophenethylamine (2C-B), 2,5-dimethoxy-4-(n)-propylthiophenethylamine (2C-T-7), 2,5-dimethoxy-4-ethylphenethylamine (2C-E, Europa), 4-iodo-2,5-dimethoxyphenethylamine (2C-I), 2,5-dimethoxy-4-ethylthiophenethylamine (2C-T-2), among others.[2,47] Phenethylamines (2C), known in the social context by several brand names, such as Erox, Nexus, Afro, Performax, Blue Mystic, T7, Beautiful, Tripstay, Tweety-Bird Mescaline, have structural similarity with SCs, catecholamines, and amphetamines and act on 5HT2A and alpha-adrenergic receptors, exerting stimulant and psychedelic effects.[2,47] Users mainly consume these substances orally (e.g., tablets, powders, pills, blotter paper), but also via injection or nasally via insufflation, commonly in combination with other drugs.[2,3,47] The recreational (e.g., dance parties, raves, nightclub) setting is the social context typical of phenethylamines (2C) use,[2] where the main motivations of use are the psychoactive effects of the drugs, as for the other stimulants/psychedelics tryptamines and piperazines.[43,46]

2.3.2. Synthetic Hallucinogens

Synthetic hallucinogens (SH) include both dissociative and hallucinogen synthetic compounds.

Hallucinogens/psychedelics include lysergamines (typically lysergic acid diethylamide [LSD]) and, as previously mentioned, tryptamines, phenethylamines, and piperazines[2,3] (for the latter groups, see also the previous sections), which produce the same effects as the traditional psychedelics mescaline and psylocibin, such as alterations of perception, mood, and cognition, through the serotoninergic system.[3,45,48] Synthetic hallucinogens (e.g., LSD derivatives, 25i-NBOMe, 4-AcO-DMT, or 2C-B) are available in the social context as pills or blotter paper, generally consumed orally, through inhalation or nasal insufflation, in recreational contexts (raves and nightclubs), with the most commonly described reasons of use being practical motives (e.g., easy alternative to LSD), although curiosity, need of self-exploration, and mystical experiences have been described as well.[3,11] Moreover, it is important to note that increasing attention also has been given to the psychedelics "micro-dosing" practice in both social and research contexts, with particular attention to LSD and psilocybin. As suggested by Kuypers and colleagues,[49] the term "micro-dosing" refers to the consumption of sub-perceptual doses, following a multiple dosing scheme with different sessions, with the aim of enhancing emotional (e.g., anxiety, stress) and mental processes.[49] Thus, such practice also has become diffuse in healthy individuals,[24] such as professionals working long hours in busy environments and students seeking performance enhancement, underscoring how this emerging trend is influencing society in several fields in parallel with the increased diffusion of IPEDs, which will be described further in a later section.

Dissociative drugs include arylcyclohexylamine and diarylethylamine products, with ketamine (brand name "Special K") and phencyclidine (PCP) (brand name "Angel Dust") having first been used for their anesthetic properties, while their designer derivatives, such as methoxetamine (MXE), 4-methoxyphencyclidine—4-MeO-PCP, 3-MeO-PCP, 2-oxo-PCE (eticyclidone), among others, have recently appeared in the recreational drug scenario.[3,50] By acting as antagonists of the N-methyl-D-aspartate (NMDA) receptor, such substances produce euphoria, depersonalization, dissociation of thought and consciousness from the body, and psychotomimetic effects, with sensory and tactile distortions,[3,50] which, in turn, are the main motivations that drive users. In fact, the typical social context for the use of dissociatives is a recreational setting, where users consume such substances in various ways (e.g., oral intake, nasal insufflation, inhalation, injection) to enjoy their psychoactive effects, driven by curiosity and the need of self-exploration.[3,11]

2.3.3. Synthetic Cannabinoid Receptor Agonists

Synthetic cannabinoids receptor agonists (SCRA), commonly known as synthetic cannabinoids, include several products chemically identified as classical cannabinoids, naphthoylindoles, carbazoles, cyclohexyl-substituted phenols, among which the following can be mentioned: JWH-018, JWH-073, JWH-398, JWH-250, CP47,497, and HU-210, among others.[2,3] SCRA are advertised as safe and legal alternatives to cannabis, with a large number of brand names (e.g., Spice, K2, Scooby Snax, Mojo, Yucatan, Geeked Up, Smacked, Fake Weed, Trippy, Bad Guy, Green Giant, Ice Dragon, AK-47); they act on cannabinoid type-1 and 2 (CB-1/2) receptors, resembling the effect of natural cannabis and Δ9-tetrahydrocannabinol.[2,3,51] Such products, sold as powder, gel, resin, capsules, and tablets, are mainly consumed by users per oral intake or smoked, using a vaporizer, and by liquid inhalation, often in combination with other substances (e.g., alcohol).[2,3,18] SCRA are reported to be mainly used for: replacing cannabis; curiosity; pragmatic reasons; their psychoactive effects, described as intense and including the feeling of "high"; seeking therapeutic effects, with the social context typical of SCRA including recreational circumstances and others (e.g., prisons, military service).[2,18,52]

2.3.4. Synthetic Depressants

Synthetic depressants include both designer opioids and hypnotics/sedatives.

Novel synthetic opioids (NSO) are a broad class of compounds acting on opiate receptors, including fentanyl- (e.g., carfentanil, ocfentanil, acetyl fentanyl, furanyl fentanyl) and not-fentanyl-analogues, such as benzamide (e.g., AH-7921, U-47700, U-77891, U-50488), piperazine, and bromadoline opioids (e.g., MT-45, W-18).[2,53,54] Among the NSOs, fentanyl-related compounds are the most diffuse. They are sold in the social context with the following brand names: Drop Dead, Serial Killer, Gray Death, and Pink, in the form of powder, adulterants mixed with heroin, or counterfeit pills resembling prescription opioids, such as hydrocodone, oxycodone, Xanax, or Norco.[2,53,54] Such designer products are consumed via a range of routes (e.g., oral intake, nasally, injection, insufflation), with the main motivations being reported as the following: pragmatic reasons, especially easy availability over the internet and even on the dark web; as substitutes for traditional opioids for opioid-abuse individuals, in light of increased restrictions on prescription opioids in the modern opioid epidemic; and self-medication of pain, sleeping problems, and anxiety.[2,3,11,53,54]

Synthetic hypnotics/sedatives, known also as designer benzodiazepines (BZD), include several products that recently appeared in the NPS scenario and which act on γ-aminobutyric acid-A (GABA-A) receptors, by resembling the action of prescription benzodiazepines.[2,3,34,55] Designer BZD, such as phenazepam, clonazolam, diclazepam, etizolam, pyrazolam, flubromazepam, flubromazolam, and alprazolam triazolobenzophenone derivative, among others, are mainly sold online as "research chemicals" or "legal benzodiazepines" and are available in several forms (e.g., powder, capsules, tablets, blotters, liquids, and pills producing "fake" versions of prescribed BZD), sometimes mixed with other substances (e.g., SCRA).[2,34,55] In the recreational scenario, users mainly consume such designer drugs orally, with other routes (e.g., intranasal, inhalation, sublingual, rectal, injection) being also described, and the main reported motives of use overlap with medical applications.[2,3,34,55] Therefore, these motivations would include pragmatic reasons; self-treatment of some conditions (e.g., withdrawal symptoms); muscle relaxant and amnesic effects; and subjective "high" perception.[2,3,34,55]

2.3.5. Gamma-hydroxybutyrate

Gamma-hydroxybutyrate (GHB), commonly known in the social context as liquid ecstasy, is a natural substance derived from GABA neurotransmitter present in the human body, especially in the central nervous system (CNS). By acting on GABA receptors, GHB exerts anxiolytic, sedative, and alcohol-mimetic actions, and it is available in salt, powder, tablet, and liquid forms, to be consumed mainly orally, by snorting or injection.[56,57] The social context typical of GHB use is the recreational setting (e.g., clubs, dance music settings), where such substance is often mixed with others and is consumed to enjoy its psychoactive effects (e.g., increased sociability, euphoria, sleep induction) or to enhance sexual performance in the context of a chem-sex event, especially among homosexual men; further, it possesses the ability to reduce weight or to enhance muscle mass, resembling anabolic agents, thus it is also used as IPED within gym community (e.g., body-builders and gym-goers),[56–58] like other image- and performance-enhancing products.

For a complete overview on motivations/patterns of NPS use, see Table 2.1.

2.3.6. Image- and Performance-Enhancing Drugs

Image- and performance-enhancing drugs (IPEDs), or "lifestyle" drugs, include a range of compounds used to boost performances in all life sectors.[59] Most IPEDs are used as fitness products, orally or injected, by athletes in elite sports, body-builders,[23] and increasingly gym-goers in the attempt to rapidly improve their physical appearance. Such products include: *anabolic-androgenic steroids* (AAS) (e.g., metandienone, methandrostenolone, stanozolol, testosterone enanthate, nandrolone, oxandrolone, drostanolone, metenolone, oxymetholone, boldenone, dehydrochloromethyltestosterone, trenbolone, mesterolone) and the peptide hormone human growth hormone (hGH), used for improving muscle mass; *hormones* (e.g., levothyroxine [T4], liothyronine [T3], designer steroids), *stimulants* and *metabolic modulators* (e.g., clenbuterol, diuretics [aldactone,] 2,4-dinitrophenol [DNP], ephedrine, caffeine) used as fat burners; *anti-estrogenic agents* (e.g., tamoxifen citrate, clomiphene citrate, letrozole); *peptide hormones* (e.g., CJC-1295, insulin growth factor [IGF], mechano growth factor [MGF], growth hormone-releasing peptide [GHRP-6], human chorionic gonadotropin [hCG]), among others.[23,60–62] Findings of a cross-sectional investigation among over 2000 exercisers across the European Union showed that 39.8% of the sample used IPEDs, with no previous medical consultation.[27]

Other types of IPEDs are used to enhance sexual performance, such as sildenafil, GHB, bremelanotide, yohimbine, and the peptide hormone skin-tanning Melanotan II,[23,57,63] to improve mood and social behavior (e.g., fluoxetine, beta-blockers, diazepam),[62] or to enhance mental performance in the academic context (e.g., methylphenidate [Ritalin]), including

Table 2.1 Main Motivations/Patterns for NPS Use in the Social Context

NPS Category	Motivation for Use	Pattern of Use
Synthetic cathinones	Practical reasons > psychopharmacological properties Replacement of other drugs Self-medication	*Route of administration*: oral, nasal, smoking, injection, rectal *Setting*: recreational context, mephedrone sessions, slamming, exchange programs involving IDU
Tryptamines	Practical reasons Recreational purpose/ psychedelic effects	*Route of administration*: oral, nasal, smoking, injection *Setting*: recreational context
Piperazines	Practical reasons Recreational purpose/ psychoactive effects IPED	*Route of administration*: oral *Setting*: recreational context
2C Phenylethylamines	Practical reasons Recreational purpose	*Route of administration*: oral, nasal, insufflation *Setting*: recreational context
Synthetic hallucinogens	Practical reasons Recreational purpose/ psychoactive effects Self-exploration IPED	*Route of administration*: oral, nasal, insufflation, intravenous *Setting*: recreational context, micro-dosing practise
Dissociatives	Practical reasons Inner exploration	*Route of administration*: oral, nasal, insufflation, inhalation, injection *Setting*: recreational context
Synthetic Cannabinoid Receptor Agonists	Practical reasons Recreational purpose Therapeutic potential	*Route of administration*: smoking, oral, inhalation *Setting*: alternative to cannabis, recreational context
Opioids	Practical reasons Replacement of other drugs Therapeutic potential	*Route of administration*: oral, nasal, insufflation, injection *Setting*: recreational context and self-chosen treatment
Sedatives/ Hypnotics	Practical reasons Self-medication	*Route of administration*: oral, sublingual, inhalation, intranasal, injection *Setting*: recreational context and self-chosen treatment
GHB	Practical reasons Recreational purpose IPED	*Route of administration*: oral, injection, snorking *Setting*: recreational context, chem-sex event, gym community

Table 2.2 Main Motivations/Patterns for IPED Use in the Social Context

Motivation for Use	IPED Category
To increase muscle mass and strength	Anabolic steroids and growth hormones
Fat burners to improve body image	Dinitrophenol (DNP), clenbuterol, ephedrine, liothyronine, levothyyroxin, diuretics
To improve skin and hair appearance	Latisse, mercury, Melanotan II
To enhance sexual performance	GHB, sildenafil, bremelanotide, yohimbine
To enhance cognitive performance	Methylphenidate, modafinil, piracetam, piperazines
To enhance mood and social behavior	Fluoxetine, beta-blockers, diazepam
All motivations listed above	Dietary/nutritional supplements

Source: Adapted from Begley et al.[23] and McVeigh et al.[62]

prescription drugs primarily used for the treatment of attention deficit hyperactivity disorder (ADHD) (e.g., atomoxetine, modafinil, prescription amphetamines such as dextroamphetamine [Adderall]), and illicit drugs (e.g., cocaine).[24,64]

Among IPEDs, a major challenge is represented by their undisclosed presence in dietary/nutritional supplements (e.g., vitamins, minerals, enzymes, herbal/botanical substances), advertised online and elsewhere as "natural and safer" alternatives to pharmaceutical products at affordable prices and in several forms (e.g., capsules, bars, powders, liquids, tablets). Their contamination has led 23 000 unaware users to the emergency room in the United Sates alone in the period between 2004 and 2013.[65] Further, Tucker and colleagues,[66] by extracting data from the FDA's Center for Drug Evaluation and Research, Tainted Products Marketed as Dietary Supplement database, were able to identify 776 adulterated dietary supplements in the period 2007–2016, with sildenafil, synthetic steroids, and sibutramine being the main reported and undisclosed adulterants.[66]

An overview on motivations/patterns for IPEDs and supplements use is provided in Table 2.2.

2.4. Conclusion

The increasing number of NPS available on the illicit drug market, in combination with the continuous emergence of new chemicals and herbal compounds, represents a serious challenge in terms of public and current regulatory responses.

In our frenetic society driven by technology and globalization and based on social media communication, with increased peer pressure to appear/perform "at the best," NPS/IPEDs use is not only diffuse in the recreational context but has become part of daily life for many individuals who do not typically consider themselves as drug users.[23] Consequently, users do not feel the need or want to receive professional help until they face an emergency. At the same time, healthcare professionals must be prepared to intervene and need to be kept up to date about the most suitable clinical strategies for both assessment and treatment. In response, various initiatives across the European Union have emerged, such as the European Drug Emergencies Network Plus (EuroDEN-Plus) for the monitoring of drug-related emergencies and the NEPTUNE clinical guidance for the Management of Acute and Chronic Harms related to NPS.[67] Despite such attempts, evidence on the efficacy of prevention programs or specific treatment for NPS use is still poor. The management would be dependent on clinical presentation, with a potential pharmacological treatment aiming to treat specific NPS-related symptoms (e.g., Naloxone in case of NSO intoxication).[53] Psychosocial interventions (PSIs) have also been suggested as potentially useful, with the NEPTUNE guidelines proposing to organize (1) brief advice/information and intervention or (2) structured drug treatment and formal psychological therapy in cases, respectively, of lower or higher NPS severity use.[67]

Evidence, however, is still inconsistent, with some authors suggesting the same strategies (e.g., harm-reduction programs, counseling) regardless of the type of NPS used,[68] while others propose more targeted interventions and encourage an integration with sexual health and substance-use services in case of comorbidity between mental health problems and NPS use.[69] Alternative prevention models, such as the theories of social norms and health beliefs, the ecology of human development, and the theory of planned behavior[70] have been proposed to prevent NPS use. However, as we have highlighted in this chapter, the need to know and better understand the underlying motivations behind NPS consumption remains the key to any type of informed solution.

In conclusion, the ever-evolving and risky NPS phenomenon needs constant monitoring to support the implementation of the most appropriate intervention strategies on several fronts, including improvement of forensic procedures and analytical methods to detect NPS and development of new forms of collaboration between research, policymaking programs, and scientific authorities. An example in this sense is given by the International Society for the Study of Emerging Drugs (ISSED) created with the scope to provide an open forum among different stakeholders and to foster collaboration and knowledge/experience exchange at the international level among multidisciplinary professionals working in the field of NPS. Only by joining efforts and developing a multiple-angle approach will we be able to better face and possibly anticipate what the next NPS trend will be.

References

1. UNODC. United Nations Office on Drugs and Crime. Global smart update 2016. 2016. https://www.unodc.org/documents/scientific/Global-SMARTUpdate-2016-vol-16.pdf.
2. Graddy R, Buresh ME, Rastegar DA. New and emerging illicit psychoactive substances. *Med Clin North Am.* 2018;102(4):697–714.
3. Shafi A, Berry AJ, Sumnall H, Wood DM, Tracy DK. New psychoactive substances: A review and updates. *Ther Adv Psychopharmacol.* 2020;10:2045125320967197. doi:10.1177/2045125320967197.
4. Assi S, Gulyamova N, Ibrahim K, Kneller P, Osselton D. Profile, effects, and toxicity of novel psychoactive substances: A systematic review of quantitative studies. *Hum Psychopharmacol Clin.* 2017;32(3):e2607.
5. Fattore L. Synthetic cannabinoids: Further evidence supporting the relationship between cannabinoids and psychosis. *Biol Psychiatry.* 2016;79(7):539–548.
6. Schifano F, Corazza O, Deluca P, et al. Psychoactive drug or mystical incense? Overview of the online available information on Spice products. *Int J Cult Ment Health.* 2009;2(2):137–144.
7. Griffiths P, Sedefov R, Gallegos A, Lopez D. How globalization and market innovation challenge how we think about and respond to drug use: "Spice," a case study. *Addiction.* 2010;105(6):951–953.
8. Zawilska JB, Andrzejczak D. Next generation of novel psychoactive substances on the horizon: A complex problem to face. *Drug Alcohol Depend.* 2015;157:1–17.
9. UNODC. Current NPS threats. March 2019. https://www.unodc.org/documents/scientific/Current_NPS_Threats_Volume_I.pdf.
10. EMCDDA. European drug report 2019: Trends and developments. 2019. http://www.emcdda.europa.eu/system/files/publications/11364/20191724_TDAT19001ENN_PDF.pdf.
11. Soussan C, Kjellgren A. The users of novel psychoactive substances: Online survey about their characteristics, attitudes and motivations. *Int J Drug Policy.* 2016;32:77–84.
12. Demant J, Bakken SA, Oksanen A, Gunnlaugsson H. Drug dealing on Facebook, Snapchat and Instagram: A qualitative analysis of novel drug markets in the Nordic countries. *Drug Alcohol Rev.* 2019;38(4):377–385.
13. Negri A, Townshend H, McSweeney T, et al. Carfentanil on the darknet: Potential scam or alarming public health threat? *Int J Drug Policy.* 2021;91:103–118.
14. Miliano C, Margiani G, Fattore L, De Luca MA. Sales and advertising channels of new psychoactive substances (NPS): Internet, social networks, and smartphone apps. *Brain Sci.* 2018;8(7):123.
15. EMCDDA. EU drug markets report. 2019. www.euda.europa.eu.
16. Barratt MJ, Cakic V, Lenton S. Patterns of synthetic cannabinoid use in Australia. *Drug Alcohol Rev.* 2013;32(2):141–146.

17. Palamar JJ, Martins SS, Su MK, Ompad DC. Self-reported use of novel psychoactive substances in a US nationally representative survey: Prevalence, correlates, and a call for new survey methods to prevent underreporting. *Drug Alcohol Depend.* 2015;156:112–119.
18. Gunderson EW, Haughey HM, Ait-Daoud N, Joshi AS, Hart CL. A survey of synthetic cannabinoid consumption by current cannabis users. *Substance Abuse.* 2014;35(2):184–189.
19. Patrick ME, O'Malley PM, Kloska DD, et al. Novel psychoactive substance use by US adolescents: Characteristics associated with use of synthetic cannabinoids and synthetic cathinones. *Drug Alcohol Rev.* 2016;35(5):586–590.
20. Soussan C, Kjellgren A. Harm reduction and knowledge exchange: A qualitative analysis of drug-related internet discussion forums. *Harm Reduct J.* 2014;11(1):25. doi:10.1186/1477-7517-11-25.
21. Werse B, Morgenstern C. How to handle legal highs? Findings from a German online survey and considerations on drug policy issues. *Drugs Alcohol Today.* 2012;12(4):222–231.
22. Vreeker A, van der Burg BG, van Laar M, Brunt TM. Characterizing users of new psychoactive substances using psychometric scales for risk-related behavior. *Addict Behav.* 2017;70:72–78.
23. Begley E, McVeigh J, Hope V, et al. *Image and Performance Enhancing Drugs: 2016 National Survey Results.* Liverpool John Moores University; 2017.
24. d'Angelo LC, Savulich G, Sahakian BJ. Lifestyle use of drugs by healthy people for enhancing cognition, creativity, motivation and pleasure. *Br J Pharmacol.* 2017;174(19):3257–3267.
25. Rabin O, Corazza O. *Emerging Drugs in Sport.* Springer; 2021.
26. Orsolini L, Papanti GD, Francesconi G, Schifano F. Mind navigators of chemicals' experimenters? A web-based description of e-psychonauts. *Cyberpsychol Behav Soc Netw.* 2015;18(5):296–300.
27. Corazza O, Simonato P, Demetrovics Z, et al. The emergence of exercise addiction, body dysmorphic disorder, and other image-related psychopathological correlates in fitness settings: A cross sectional study. *PLoS One.* 2019;14(4):e0213060.
28. di Giannantonio M, Negri A, Schiavone S, et al. Prescription drug misuse in "clubbers" and disco goers in Ibiza. *Front Psychiatry.* 2020;11:592–594.
29. Krupski A, Graves MC, Bumgardner K, Roy-Byrne P. Comparison of homeless and non-homeless problem drug users recruited from primary care safety-net clinics. *J Subst Abuse Treat.* 2015;58:84–89.
30. Ramanathan S, McCurdy CR. Kratom (*Mitragyna speciosa*): Worldwide issues. *Curr Opin Psychiatry.* 2020;33(4):312–318.
31. Prevete E, Hupli A, Marrinan S, et al. Exploring the use of kratom (*Mitragyna speciosa*) via the YouTube data tool: A novel netnographic analysis. *Emerg Trends Drugs Addict Health.* 2021;1:100007.
32. Bersani G, Prevete E. Novel psychoactive substances (NPS) use in severe mental illness (SMI) patients: Potential changes in the phenomenology of psychiatric diseases. *Hum Psychopharmacol.* 2017;32(3). doi:10.1002/hup.2591.
33. Marrinan S, Roman-Urrestarazu A, Naughton D, et al. Hair analysis for the detection of drug use: Is there potential for evasion? *Hum Psychopharmacol.* 2017;32(3). doi:10.1002/hup.2587.
34. Zawilska JB, Wojcieszak J. An expanding world of new psychoactive substances-designer benzodiazepines. *Neurotoxicology.* 2019;73:8–16.
35. UNODC. World Drug Report 2016. 2016. https://www.unodc.org/doc/wdr2016/WORLD_DRUG_REPORT_2016_web.pdf.
36. Mazurkiewicz MR, Glogowski M, Mrowińska D, Pakulski M, Matyjaszczyk M, Kardas P. [Prevalence, reasons, and forms of use of legal highs by internet-based survey participants]. *Psychiatr Pol.* 2013;47(6):1143–1155.
37. Corazza O, Simonato P, Corkery J, Trincas G, Schifano F. "Legal highs": Safe and legal "heavens"? A study on the diffusion, knowledge and risk awareness of novel psychoactive drugs among students in the UK. *Riv Psichiatr.* 2014;49(2):89–94.

38. Dubey MJ, Ghosh R, Chatterjee S, Biswas P, Chatterjee S, Dubey S. COVID-19 and addiction. *Diabetes Metab Syndr.* 2020;14(5):817–823.
39. Rajkumar RP. COVID-19 and mental health: A review of the existing literature. *Asian J Psychiatry.* 2020;52:102066.
40. Pieprzyca E, Skowronek R, Nižnanský Ľ, Czekaj P. Synthetic cathinones: From natural plant stimulant to new drug of abuse. *Eur J Pharmacol.* 2020;875:173012.
41. Péterfi A, Tarján A, Horváth GC, Csesztregi T, Nyírády A. Changes in patterns of injecting drug use in Hungary: A shift to synthetic cathinones. *Drug Test Anal.* 2014;6(7–8):825–831.
42. German CL, Fleckenstein AE, Hanson GR. Bath salts and synthetic cathinones: An emerging designer drug phenomenon. *Life Sci.* 2014;97(1):2–8.
43. Welz A, Koba M. Piperazine derivatives as dangerous abused compounds. *Acta Pharm.* 2020;70(4):423–441.
44. Katz DP, Deruiter J, Bhattacharya D, et al. Benzylpiperazine: "A messy drug." *Drug Alcohol Depend.* 2016;164:1–7.
45. Araújo AM, Carvalho F, Bastos Mde L, Guedes de Pinho P, Carvalho M. The hallucinogenic world of tryptamines: An updated review. *Arch Toxicol.* 2015;89(8):1151–1173.
46. Tittarelli R, Mannocchi G, Pantano F, Romolo FS. Recreational use, analysis and toxicity of tryptamines. *Curr Neuropharmacol.* 2015;13(1):26–46.
47. Dean BV, Stellpflug SJ, Burnett AM, Engebretsen KM. 2C or not 2C: Phenethylamine designer drug review. *J Med Toxicol.* 2013;9(2):172–178.
48. Nichols DE. Psychedelics. *Pharmacol Rev.* 2016;68(2):264–355.
49. Kuypers KP, Ng L, Erritzoe D, et al. Microdosing psychedelics: More questions than answers? An overview and suggestions for future research. *J Psychopharmacol.* 2019;33(9):1039–1057.
50. Tamama K, Lynch MJ. Newly emerging drugs of abuse. In: Nader MA, Hurd YL, eds. *Substance Use Disorders: From Etiology to Treatment.* Springer International; 2020:463–502.
51. Castaneto MS, Gorelick DA, Desrosiers NA, Hartman RL, Pirard S, Huestis MA. Synthetic cannabinoids: Epidemiology, pharmacodynamics, and clinical implications. *Drug Alcohol Depend.* 2014;144:12–41.
52. Corazza O, Coloccini S, Marrinan S, et al. Novel psychoactive substances in custodial settings: A mixed method investigation on the experiences of people in prison and professionals working with them. *Front Psychiatry.* 2020;11:460.
53. Armenian P, Vo KT, Barr-Walker J, Lynch KL. Fentanyl, fentanyl analogs and novel synthetic opioids: A comprehensive review. *Neuropharmacology.* 2018;134:121–132.
54. Beardsley PM, Zhang Y. Synthetic opioids. *Handb Exp Pharmacol.* 2018;252:353–381.
55. Orsolini L, Corkery JM, Chiappini S, et al. New/designer benzodiazepines: An analysis of the literature and psychonauts' trip reports. *Curr Neuropharmacol.* 2020;18(9):809–837.
56. Corkery JM, Loi B, Claridge H, et al. Gamma hydroxybutyrate (GHB), gamma butyrolactone (GBL) and 1,4-butanediol (1,4-BD; BDO): A literature review with a focus on UK fatalities related to non-medical use. *Neurosci Biobehav Rev.* 2015;53:52–78.
57. Kapitány-Fövény M, Mervó B, Corazza O, et al. Enhancing sexual desire and experience: An investigation of the sexual correlates of gamma-hydroxybutyrate (GHB) use. *Hum Psychopharmacol Clin.* 2015;30(4):276–284.
58. Brennan R, Van Hout MC. Gamma-hydroxybutyrate (GHB): A scoping review of pharmacology, toxicology, motives for use, and user groups. *J Psychoact Drugs.* 2014;46(3):243–251.
59. McVeigh J, Evans-Brown M, Bellis MA. Human enhancement drugs and the pursuit of perfection. *Adicciones.* 2012;24(3):185–190.
60. McVeigh J, Begley E. Anabolic steroids in the UK: An increasing issue for public health. *Drugs Educ Prev Policy.* 2017;24(3):278–285.

61. Shimko KM, Piatkowski T, Thomas KV, et al. Performance- and image-enhancing drug use in the community: Use prevalence, user demographics and the potential role of wastewater-based epidemiology. *J Hazard Mater.* 2021;419:126340.
62. McVeigh J, Chandler M, Yarwood GA. Exercise and the use of image & performance enhancing drugs within the gym environment. 2023:121–136.
63. Brennan R, Wells JG, Van Hout MC. An unhealthy glow? A review of melanotan use and associated clinical outcomes. *Perform Enhance Health.* 2014;3(2):78–92.
64. Hildt E, Lieb K, Franke AG. Life context of pharmacological academic performance enhancement among university students: A qualitative approach. *BMC Med Ethics.* 2014;15:23. doi:10.1186/1472-6939-15-23.
65. Geller AI, Shehab N, Weidle NJ, et al. Emergency department visits for adverse events related to dietary supplements. *N Engl J Med.* 2015;373(16):1531–1540.
66. Tucker J, Fischer T, Upjohn L, Mazzera D, Kumar M. Unapproved pharmaceutical ingredients included in dietary supplements associated with US Food and Drug Administration warnings. *JAMA Netw Open.* 2018;1(6):e183337.
67. Abdulrahim D, Bowden-Jones O, NEPTUNE Expert Group. *Guidance on the Management of Acute and Chronic Harms of Club Drugs and Novel Psychoactive Substances.* Novel Psychoactive Treatment UK Network (NEPTUNE); 2015.
68. Tracy DK, Wood DM, Baumeister D. Novel psychoactive substances: Types, mechanisms of action, and effects. *BMJ.* 2017;356:i6848.
69. Ralphs R, Gray P. New psychoactive substances: new service provider challenges. *Drugs Educ Prevent Policy.* 2018;25(4):301–312.
70. Kempf C, Llorca P-M, Pizon F, Brousse G, Flaudias V. What's new in addiction prevention in young people: A literature review of the last years of research. *Front Psychol.* 2017;8:1131. doi:10.3389/fpsyg.2017.01131.

3

Analytical and Biochemical Evaluation of New Psychoactive Substances

Jürg Gertsch

3.1. Introduction

Human curiosity and the drive for innovation have stimulated the search for psychoactive substances throughout history, from the exploration of natural sources in prehistoric times to the systematic synthesis of natural product-inspired or entirely novel molecules in the early 20th century. These initial efforts have given rise to a wide range of prototype stimulants, sedatives, narcotics, and psychedelics.[1,2] However, every year, dozens of new psychoactive substances (NPS) are being reported, which are used without prior toxicity assessments or a thorough understanding of their mechanisms of action, posing significant risks to consumers.[3] NPS are often slight modifications of existing psychoactive drugs, avoiding their classification under drug-control laws, which is why they are sometimes referred to as "legal highs." Although some of these substances, such as bupropion (a substituted cathinone) or nabilone, a (−)-trans-Δ^9-tetrahydrocannabinol (THC) derivative, have been developed into approved drugs, most reported psychoactive substances remain classified as NPS *sensu stricto* and are not listed in drug schedules or controlled substances laws.[4] For example, the large-scale production of purified cannabinoids, including cannabidiol, has led to the frequent emergence of new semisynthetic THC-like molecules, with new variants appearing online each year.[5] The United Nations Office on Drugs and Crime (UNODC) defines NPS as substances of abuse, either in pure form or as preparations, that are not controlled under the 1961 Single Convention on Narcotic Drugs or the 1971 Convention on Psychotropic Substances but that may pose a public health threat. The United States Controlled Substances

Act (CSA) considers NPS to fall under the Federal Analogue Act if they are chemically and pharmacologically like a controlled substance and are intended for human consumption, thereby subjecting them to regulation as controlled substances. The European Community combines a centralized framework, including the Early Warning System (EWS) and rapid risk assessment by the European Monitoring Centre for Drugs and Drug Addiction (EMCDDA), with national measures to control NPS.

Before reviewing recent methodological developments for detecting and assaying NPS in the laboratory (i.e., analytically or preclinically), it is important to note the diverse sources of NPS. Intrigued by the neuropharmacological effects of psychoactive substances, ranging from euphoria, relaxation, hallucinations, heightened energy, and enhanced sensory perception to empathy, yet also mindful of their potential aversive impacts, especially psychosis, *Homo sapiens* has long walked a delicate line between the creation and consumption of substances that can be both beneficial and harmful. Clearly, many NPS are associated with severe health risks, including overdoses, organ damage, addiction, and mental health issues.[6] The lack of comprehensive data on long-term effects makes their use particularly concerning and highlights the need for systematic and fast preclinical assessment. Substances once exclusively used by healers in ritual contexts to interact with the supernatural world have now become a profane, often hedonistic, playground for curious adolescents and recreational drug seekers. This problematic shift partly explains the booming success of smart shops in countries where psychoactive substances are legally sold, such as the Netherlands and Portugal. Polytoxicomaniacs, those who experiment with multiple substances, freely test NPS and share their subjective (i.e., anecdotal) experiences in social media and internet fora. These "chemohackers" actively seek novel ways to alter consciousness, blending published technological innovation with exploratory drug use.[7] Not surprisingly, today NPS are inspired largely by information available on the internet. A noteworthy example of a science-inspired NPS is the smoking of liverworts (*Radula* spp.) containing cannabinoid-like perrottetines, which are weak psychoactive THC-like natural products that activate cannabinoid CB1 receptors.[8] These liverworts have not previously been known to be psychoactive, and their use was inspired by scientific reports on the cannabinoid-like natural products they contain.

Historically, psychoactive natural products of ethnopharmacological value, such as morphine, cocaine, mescaline, psilocybin, dimethyltryptamine, mitragynine, and cathinones, among many others, have been isolated, synthesized, and studied extensively, eventually leading to the elucidation of their molecular mechanisms of action and thus understanding of their pharmacological effects.[9] These structurally relatively simple molecules have inspired synthetic chemists to develop derivatives, many of which exhibit similar or even opposing effects. For instance, the μ-opioid receptor (MOR) antagonistic properties of naloxone compared to the agonistic effects of morphine highlight how minor chemical modifications (specifically, replacing 2 hydroxyl groups with an allyl and a keto group) can profoundly transform pharmacological outcomes. THC, a partial CB1 cannabinoid receptor agonist from cannabis, inspired the synthesis of more potent CB1 receptor full agonists; the emergence of these highly potent synthetic cannabinoid NPS revealed for the first time the severe toxic effects mediated by full CB1 receptor activation, culminating in the "Zombie outbreak" in New York in 2016.[10] While neuropharmacologists today are confronted with the challenge of how to rapidly and efficiently detect and classify NPS without the need to go into human trials, NPS cannot be discussed without the human experience. The pioneering work of American biochemist Alexander Shulgin (1925–2014) represents the most significant example on the non-clinical study of psychoactive substances and NPS.[2] Driven by curiosity, Shulgin synthesized and personally tested over 200 novel phenethylamines and tryptamines, meticulously documenting his findings in the influential books *PiHKAL* (*Phenethylamines I Have Known and Loved*) (1991) and *TiHKAL* (*Tryptamines I Have Known and Loved*) (1997).[11,12] During that era, systematic biochemical and analytical profiling of these substances was not yet possible as receptors and biochemical systems in the central nervous system (CNS) had only started to be uncovered.

In the late 1990s, as a PhD student at ETH (*Eidgenössische Technische Hochschule*, or Swiss Federal Institute of Technology) Zurich, I was intrigued by reports about the unique, short, and intense hallucinogenic effects of the "sage of the diviners" (*Salvia divinorum*). At that time, neither the plant nor the constituents were regulated in Switzerland. Bryan Roth's research group and collaborators were among the first to more systematically employ biochemical assays on neurotransmitter receptors to identify ligand interactions of NPS. In 2002, the discovery that salvinorin A is a potent and selective kappa opioid receptor (KOR) agonist[13] was groundbreaking and underscored the value of receptor-based biochemical assays in understanding psychoactive substances. Together with the insight that the hallucinogen muscimol, the

Table 3.1 Molecular Targets of Major NPS Classes

NPS Class	Molecular Mechanisms/Targets
Synthetic opioids	*Endorphin system, opioid receptors*
Synthetic cannabinoids	*Endocannabinoid system, cannabinoid receptors*
Synthetic cathinones	*Monoamine transporters (NET, DAT, SERT)*
Amphetamine-type stimulants	*Monoamine transporters (NET, DAT, SERT, VMAT2)*
Benzodiazepine analogues	*GABA(A) receptors, CB1 receptor, opioid receptors*
Phenetylamines, tryptamines	*Serotonin receptors (5-HT2A)*
Piperazines	*Monoamine receptors*
Other hallucinogens	*Cholinergic system, ion channels, KOR, GABA(A)*
Arylcyclohexamines	*NMDA glutamate receptors*

psychoactive component in fly agaric (*Amanita muscaria*), mimics the neurotransmitter GABA and binds to the same binding site in GABA receptors,[14] the case of salvinorin A supported the theory that psychoactive substances exert their effect through pharmacodynamic effects integrating potency and kinetics of neurotransmitter interactions. Advancements in receptor biochemistry and assay development have since revolutionized the profiling of psychoactive substances. Today, we know that a large group of hallucinogens (the classical serotonergic psychedelics) all interact and partially activate specific serotonin receptors, in particular the serotonin receptor 5HT2A.[15] Thus, receptor interaction signatures trigger specific neuropharmacological effects. A limited number of known receptor systems can mediate the majority of specific psychoactive effects of NPS (Table 3.1).

Similarly, analytical developments, particularly liquid chromatography mass spectrometry (LC-MS)- or gas chromatography mass spectrometry (GC-MS)-based methods and molecular networking (MN) approaches, have significantly enhanced our ability to screen for NPS based on their chemical structures and similarities. Validated animal assays facilitate the rapid pharmacological characterization of NPS and allow for routine preclinical pharmacotoxicological assessments.

An understanding of the molecular identity and biochemical and receptor-mediated pharmacological mechanisms of these substances is critical for informing legal classification, scheduling, and harm-reduction strategies.[6] In this chapter, I will review the analytical tools to detect known and likely NPS using spectrometric and spectroscopic methods, the progress made in experimentally measuring and predicting receptor interactions of psychoactive substances using *in silico* tools, as well as versatile animal assays.

3.2. Analytical Tools: More Accurate, More Sensitive

Developments in chemical analytics, which is the qualitative and quantitative analysis of chemical substances to determine their composition, structure, properties, and interactions have dramatically impacted NPS research.[16] Today, technological advancements match the need for routine screening of NPS based on the legal frameworks (Figure 3.1). In particular, LC-MS-based methodologies and molecular networking (*vide infra*) have changed our routine toolbox to screen for NPS.[17]

Today, more than 800 NPS and regulated psychoactive substances are being monitored by official agencies, which poses a challenge to routine analytics. Shafi et al.[18] highlight the limited availability of timely clinical testing for NPS toxicity during acute presentations, recommending that diagnoses be based primarily on clinical features. However, NPS toxidromes are often nonspecific (e.g., synthetic stimulants or cannabinoids), and users may ingest multiple substances, complicating identification. NPS identification is not only relevant from a forensic point of view, but also for physicians treating patients who consume NPS. Simple standardized analytical methods like colorimetric tests, immunoassays, and mass spectrometry are used for NPS detection in drug matrices, but most tests identify only a limited number of compound types. Colorimetric tests are portable and easy to use but have significant drawbacks, including user variability, cross-reactivity, and limited coverage of NPS compounds. Moreover, commercially available immunoassays are limited to testing for relatively small selections of NPS. A study of cross-reactivity among commercially available immunoassay kits reported failure to detect certain NPS samples tested.[19] Therefore, to unambiguously identify an NPS for forensic purposes from drug or consumer matrices requires through high-precision analytics, which generally involves hyphenated methods coupled to mass spectrometry or spectroscopic methods like nuclear magnetic resonance (NMR).

Traditional matrices like whole blood, plasma, serum, and urine are widely used in toxicological analyses and are regarded as the standard. However, growing research has explored alternative matrices for drug screening, with oral fluid and hair[20] gaining popularity for various toxicological applications. Moreover, NPS can be detected and monitored in wastewaters.[21] Unfortunately, data on concentration ranges for the different NPS classes in biological matrices are mostly incomplete and/or missing, which creates a need for pharmacokinetics and tissue-distribution studies

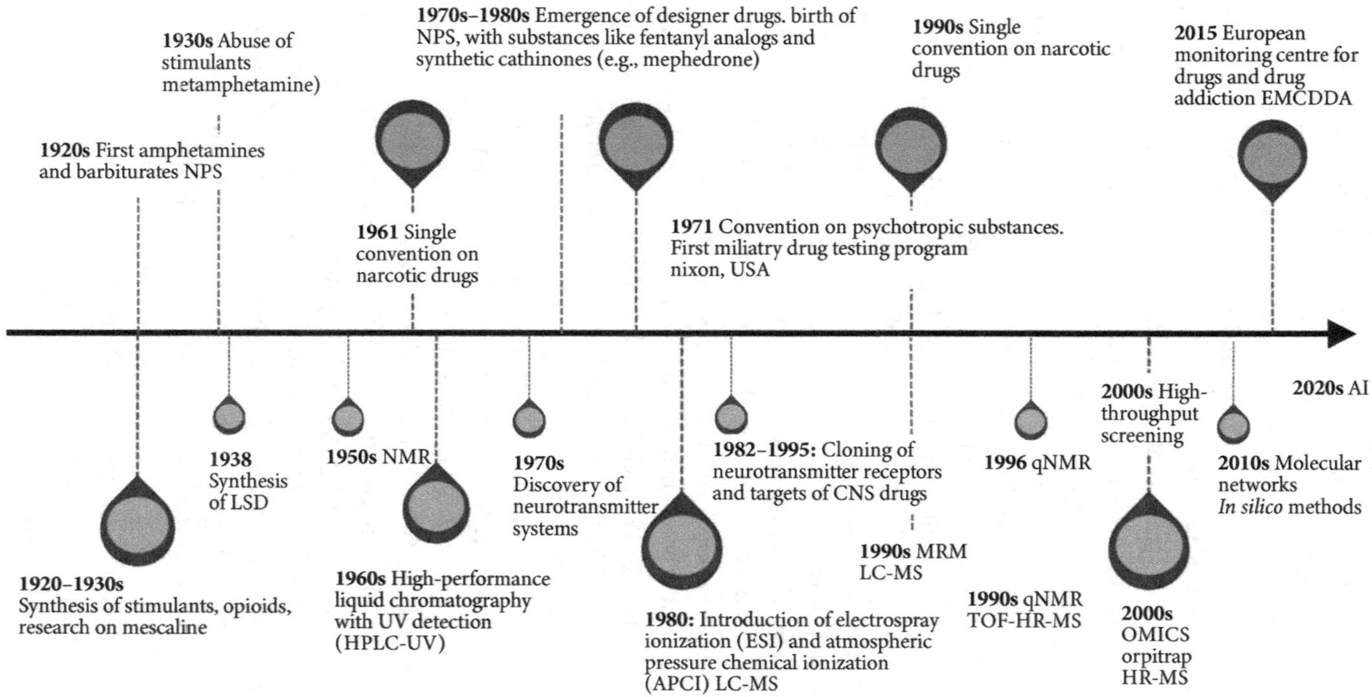

Figure 3.1. Timeline of the emergence and regulation of NPS with technological and methodological advancements in analytics and biochemistry.

in preclinical animal models, as well as from human blood samples. Gameli et al.[22] have provided a comprehensive review on designer benzodiazepines, emphasizing the need for research focusing on NPS metabolite identification. Extracting NPS and their metabolites from diverse matrices can be challenging and requires standardized and refined methods prior to analysis.[23] The preanalytical handling and extraction methodologies can impact the identification and quantification of NPS. NMR has the advantage that samples do not need to undergo chromatographic separation. As reviewed by Prates Serrano et al.,[24] quantitative ^{1}H NMR (^{1}H-qNMR) is a feasible methodology to identify and quantify NPS, especially in the absence of certified reference materials (CRM). As pointed out by Graziano et al.,[25] new screening and sensitive targeted methods for NPS and their metabolites should be developed in different types of biological matrices, where concentration of substances and matrix effects can be different. Castaing-Cordier et al.[26] developed a workflow in which the elucidation of different NPS is assisted with databases without the exact mass, combining 1D and 2D NMR measurements on a benchtop spectrometer with infrared (IR) spectroscopy. While NMR can correctly annotate atoms and elucidate absolute structures and stereochemistry, mass spectrometry is highly sensitive and versatile. The most frequently used methods in NPS detection and identification are thus based on LC-MS or GC-MS. The applications of high-resolution mass spectrometry (HRMS) for the analysis of NPS in forensic drug chemistry and analytical toxicology has been reviewed by Pasin et al.[27] For forensic purposes, the use of GC-MS/MS or LC-MS/MS to perform multiple reaction monitoring (MRM) for the quantification, using high-sensitivity triple quadrupole systems (QTRAP), is state of the art. As comprehensively reviewed by Klingberg et al.,[23] techniques like MRM and first level mass spectrometry (MS1) monitoring of pseudomolecular ions are commonly used in drug screening, and while being optimal for quantification, these techniques offer limited structural insights and are less effective for identifying unknown compounds. Given the dynamic and unpredictable nature of the NPS market, non-targeted analytical approaches are becoming more important. For instance, Krajewski et al.[28] described a method utilizing a quadrupole time-of-flight (QTOF) instrument in data-dependent acquisition (DDA) mode to identify emerging synthetic opioids. While DDA enables the detection of unknown compounds, it may overlook analytes present at low concentrations relative to the sample matrix.

In contrast, data-independent acquisition (DIA) techniques support both targeted library-based screening and nontargeted analyses through advanced data interpretation. One variation, variable DIA, segments the full mass-to-charge (m/z) range into smaller, sequentially analyzed windows, reducing noise in extracted ion chromatograms (EICs) by limiting the number of precursor ions fragmented per window.[29] Salomone et al.[30] showcased the use of Sequential Windowed Acquisition of All Theoretical Fragment Ion Mass Spectra (SWATH™) to detect fentanyl analogues and their metabolites in hair samples, employing 12 mass windows spanning m/z 230–450. A strategy is identifying NPS and their metabolites, utilizing diagnostic common fragments and neutral losses specific to each NPS chemical core. This approach builds on the framework outlined by Niessen,[31] which detailed the fragmentation patterns of traditional drugs using positive-ion LC-MS/MS. Mardal et al.[32] demonstrated that 10 selected NPS, analyzed using 4 different MS instruments under similar collision energy conditions, consistently produced the same qualitative fragment ions. Although the experiment was limited by sample dilution and instrument dynamic range, the authors suggested that identifying NPS based on the qualitative comparison of m/z values for diagnostic fragments and precursor ions could serve as a reliable preliminary identification method. Building on this finding, they developed HighResNPS (https://highresnps.com/), a concise, user-friendly database designed for forensic laboratories to share MS data on NPS. The database includes molecular formulas, exact masses of precursor ions, and diagnostic fragment ions, facilitating collaborative identification efforts. The noteworthy NPS-MS is a web server (https://nps-ms.ca/) that predicts MS/MS spectra for NPS compounds and identifies them by comparing against a database of ~8.7 million predicted NPS compounds and 24.5 million ESI-QToF-MS/MS spectra.[33] The importance of a dual targeted/untargeted data-mining strategy for metabolite identification of NPS has been exemplified with 3F-α-pyrrolydinovalerophenone.[34]

3.3. NPS Molecular Networks

Molecular networking (MN) is a computational strategy that may help visualization and interpretation of the complex data arising from MS analysis. MN can identify potential similarities among all MS/MS spectra within the dataset and to propagate annotation to unknown but related molecules.[35] This approach exploits the assumption that structurally related molecules produce similar fragmentation patterns, and therefore they should be related within a network.[36] In MN, MS/MS data are represented in a graphical form, where each node represents an ion with an associated fragmentation spectrum; the links among the nodes indicate similarities of the spectra. By propagation of the structural information within the network, unknown but structurally related molecules can be highlighted and successful dereplication can be obtained;[37] this may be particularly useful for metabolite and NPS identification. MN is increasingly being used in NPS research and as a useful tool. In their study, Vincenti et al.[38] used MN to successfully identify unexpected fentanyl analogues in 2 drug seizures, revealing the value of this method in analyzing NPS. By employing liquid chromatography-high resolution mass spectrometry (LC-HRMS) and the Global Natural Product Search (GNPS) platform, the team identified and connected synthetic cannabinoids and fentanyl derivatives within molecular networks. Analyses of seized materials and biological samples further demonstrated the utility of the MN strategy in identifying closely related compounds and metabolites of synthetic cannabinoids.[39]

3.4. Experimental Biochemical Assays and *In Silico* Tools

Most NPS have major targets but also show some degree of polypharmacology. Currently, targets can be classified into receptor groups (Table 3.1). With the identification of most targets of NPS and the emergence of medium-throughput assays to measure ligand receptor interactions in vitro, the characterization of NPS has become easier in recent decades. Companies and contract research organizations, including Eurofins®, Revvity®, XenoTech®, Retrogenix®, and many others, offer services to rationally profile small molecules on all known major receptors. The effects of NPS can be easily assessed by automated fluorescent-based methods like FLIPR assays,[40] or in patch-clamp experiments.[41] In recent years, G protein-coupled receptor (GPCR) high-throughput screening (HTS) not only has led to the identification of new and repurposing of existing drugs, and the deorphanization of GPCRs with unknown ligands,[42] but also is becoming a routine tool to screen NPS. To date, relatively few laboratories specialize in identifying the molecular targets of NPS.

In silico tools have become invaluable in the prediction and study of NPS and their interactions with the CNS. These computational methods include molecular modeling, machine learning, and cheminformatics to uncover the structure-activity relationships (SAR) of various compounds. By simulating the interactions between potential NPS and CNS receptors, such as neurotransmitter transporters, ion channels, or G-protein coupled receptors, predictions about the mode of action can be made.[43] Through ligand pharmacophore similarity searches, potential pharmacological effects or polypharmacological relationships can be predicted.[44] Additionally, *in silico* methods allow for the prediction of binding affinities, offering a rational estimation of how strongly a compound might bind to specific CNS receptors. Such predictions provide an early indication of a substance's psychoactive potency and potential therapeutic or recreational use, but need to be confirmed experimentally. Beyond predicting activity, *in silico* tools also help assess critical properties such as toxicity and ADMET (absorption, distribution, metabolism, excretion, and toxicity) profiles.[45] This is particularly important for NPS, as many are consumed without any prior evaluation of their safety or long-term effects. By identifying potential risks and off-target interactions, these methods contribute to harm reduction and guide the prioritization of substances for experimental validation. By combining computational predictions with experimental data, scientists can better understand the pharmacology of NPS and their impact on the CNS while minimizing costs and risks. In summary, *in silico* tools are increasingly relevant for modern NPS research. The ability to predict interactions, assess risks, and guide discovery makes them indispensable in uncovering the complex pharmacology of NPS and their effects on the CNS.

3.5. The Use of Animal Models to Study NPS

Since it is impossible to simulate neuropharmacological effects in a petri dish without an *in vivo* context, the use of animal models to study psychoactive substances, including NPS, is intuitive and well established (Figure 3.2). Moreover, NPS often exhibit highly diverse chemical structures and pharmacological profiles, making it difficult to get data from established standardized dosing and testing protocols from the non-controlled use in humans. Animal models are indispensable because the rapid emergence of NPS outpaces the understanding of their pharmacological and possible

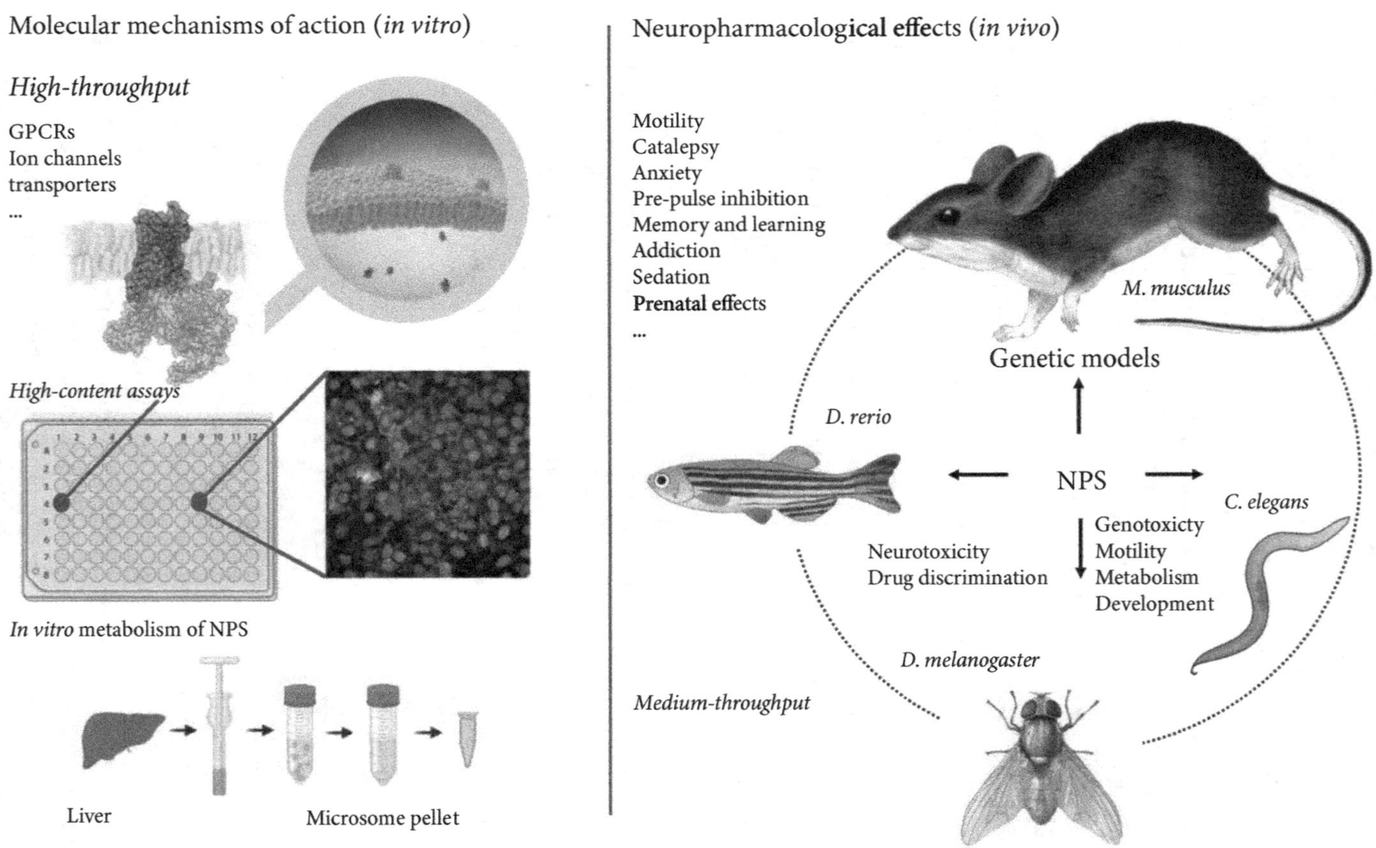

Figure 3.2. Preclinical biochemical assays in vitro and animal models help to profile NPS and allow for systematic comparative pharmacotoxicological assessments.

toxicological effects, leaving critical gaps in understanding how NPS work. Although animal models have limited value to predict therapeutic effects in humans and are only of limited use for de novo CNS drug discovery,[46] they remain essential for elucidating the mechanisms of action and potential risks. Importantly, animal models provide a controlled environment to assess dose-dependent acute and chronic effects, offering insights that are difficult to obtain otherwise.

Different model organisms have been proposed to be suitable assays for NPS, ranging from worms to rodents.[47] While the usefulness of the small nematode *Caenorhabditis elegans* and the fruit fly *Drosophila melanogaster* to assess the neuropharmacological effects of NPS remains questionable, these versatile and ethically unproblematic animal models may offer valuable tools for comparative toxicological studies.[48] *C. elegans* has many conserved genes involved in neurotransmission, including enzymes, transporters, and receptors, and thus offers a possible model for NPS testing.[49] We have shown that *C. elegans* expresses cannabinoid receptor orthologs that interact with cannabinoids.[50] Moreover, *C. elegans* may be a feasible simple animal model for identifying molecular mechanisms of addiction, including opioid addiction.[51] This worm has been successfully used to study the sedative and anxiolytic effects of kavalactones, which are in part mediated by effects on neuromuscular transmission.[52] Fruit flies exposed to drugs of abuse during different developmental stages, such as larvae and adults, exhibit molecular, morphological, behavioral, and survival changes that are dependent on the dosage. These phenotypes resemble the adverse effects of psychoactive substances in clinical medicine.[53]

Zebrafish (*Danio rerio*), which are relatively easy to handle and are optimal for pharmatoxicological screening,[54] have been used to study different NPS. Kawahara et al.[55] reported that the designer hallucinogen 25B-NBOMe recapitulates serotonin receptor-dependent rhabdomyolysis in zebrafish larvae. Since different NPS, including benzodiazepines, have been shown to lead to rhabdomyolysis, this in vivo assay offers a simple screening platform. However, when it comes to CNS effects, commonalities and differences of mammalian versus the fish model pose significant problems,[56] also considering the different ADMET properties of NPS in fish versus mammals. Nevertheless, the effects of fentanyl on zebrafish larvae and metabolism were shown to be similar to rodents, supporting the hypothesis of using zebrafish larvae as a suitable rapid screening tool to investigate opioid NPS.[57]

From a scientific perspective, mice offer interesting animal models as genetic manipulation, such as knock-outs or knock-ins, allow proof-of-principle studies related to the molecular mechanisms of action of NPS. The combination of in vitro receptor studies with genetic and pharmacological studies in vivo is a powerful tool to profile the mechanisms of action of NPS.

3.6. Conclusions

Diverse analytical methods, ranging from simple colorimetric tests to high-end spectroscopic and spectrometric quantitative analyses, today allow for a precise identification and quantification of NPS in different matrices, even in the absence of CRM. The technological breakthroughs of the past 2 decades, including HTS and *in silico* ligand similarity and receptor docking studies and animal studies, have facilitated insights into receptor interactions and the biochemical effects of NPS (Figure 3.2), enabling more precise evaluation of their potential pharmacotoxicological properties in the laboratory. While there is a demand for easily accessible assays to screen and identify NPS, highly specialized spectrometric and spectroscopic methods are increasingly becoming available to identify known and possible NPS and their metabolites from human samples. A major challenge for global NPS research is the limited availability of these high-end, cost-intensive instruments in developing countries, highlighting the urgent need to develop simple, cost-effective assays to bridge this gap.

References

1. King LA, Kicman AT. A brief history of "new psychoactive substances." *Drug Test Anal.* 2011;3(7–8):401–403. doi:10.1002/dta.319.
2. Appendino G, Minassi A, Taglialatela-Scafati O. Recreational drug discovery: Natural products as lead structures for the synthesis of smart drugs. *Nat Prod Rep.* 2014;31(7):880–904.
3. Peacock A, Bruno R, Gisev N, et al. New psychoactive substances: Challenges for drug surveillance, control, and public health responses. *Lancet.* 2019 Nov 2;394(10209):1668–1684. doi:10.1016/S0140-6736(19)32231-7.
4. Neicun J, Roman-Urrestarazu A, Czabanowska K. Legal responses to novel psychoactive substances implemented by ten European countries: An analysis from legal epidemiology. *Emerg Trends Drugs Addict Health.* 2022;2:100044. doi:10.1016/j.etdah.2022.100044.
5. Caprari C, Ferri E, Vandelli MA, Citti C, Cannazza G. An emerging trend in novel psychoactive substances (NPSs): Designer THC. *J Cannabis Res.* 2024 May 3;6(1):21. doi:10.1186/s42238-024-00226-y.

6. Mohr ALA, Logan BK, Fogarty MF, et al. Reports of adverse events associated with use of novel psychoactive substances, 2017–2020: A review. *J Anal Toxicol.* 2022 Jul 14;46(6):e116–e185. doi:10.1093/jat/bkac023.
7. Baumeister D, Tojo LM, Tracy DK. Legal highs: Staying on top of the flood of novel psychoactive substances. *Ther Adv Psychopharmacol.* 2015;5(2):97–132. doi:10.1177/2045125314559539.
8. Chicca A, Schafroth MA, Reynoso-Moreno I, et al. Uncovering the psychoactivity of a cannabinoid from liverworts associated with a legal high. *Sci Adv.* 2018;4(10):eaat2166. doi:10.1126/sciadv.aat2166.
9. Skalicka-Wozniak K, Gertsch J. Antipsychotic natural products. *Annu Rep Med Chem.* 2020;55:481–515. doi:10.1016/bs.armc.2020.03.004.
10. Adams AJ, Banister SD, Irizarry L, et al. "Zombie" outbreak caused by the synthetic cannabinoid AMB-FUBINACA in New York. *N Engl J Med.* 2017;376(3):235–242.
11. Shulgin A, Shulgin A. *PiHKAL: A Chemical Love Story.* Transform Press; 1991.
12. Shulgin A, Shulgin A. *TiHKAL: The Continuation.* Transform Press; 1997.
13. Roth BL, Baner K, Westkaemper R, et al. Salvinorin A: a potent naturally occurring nonnitrogenous kappa opioid selective agonist. *Proc Natl Acad Sci U S A.* 2002 Sep;99(18):11934–11939. doi: 10.1073/pnas.182234399.
14. Johnston GA. Muscimol as an ionotropic GABA receptor agonist. *Neurochem Res.* 2014 Oct;39(10):1942–1947. doi:10.1007/s11064-014-1245-y.
15. Nichols DE. Hallucinogens. *Pharmacol Ther.* 2004 Feb;101(2):131–181. doi:10.1016/j.pharmthera.2003.11.002.
16. Wagmann L, Maurer HH. Bioanalytical methods for new psychoactive substances. *Handb Exp Pharmacol.* 2018;252:413–439.
17. Feigel B, Adamowicz P, Wybraniec S. Recent advances in analysis of new psychoactive substances by means of liquid chromatography coupled with low-resolution tandem mass spectrometry. *Anal Bioanal Chem.* 2024 Jan;416(1):107–124. doi:10.1007/s00216-023-05057-z.
18. Shafi A, Berry AJ, Sumnall H, Wood DM, Tracy DK. New psychoactive substances: A review and updates. *Ther Adv Psychopharmacol.* 2020;10:2045125320967197. doi:10.1177/2045125320967197.
19. Cieri G, Mohr ALA, Mastrovito R, Logan BK. Evaluating cross-reactivity of new psychoactive substances (NPS) in human whole blood by enzyme-linked immunosorbent assay (ELISA). *J Anal Toxicol.* 2024 Mar 28;48(3):191–196. doi:10.1093/jat/bkac023.
20. Kyriakou C, Pellegrini M, García-Algar O, Marinelli E, Zaami S. Recent trends in analytical methods to determine new psychoactive substances in hair. *Curr Neuropharmacol.* 2017;15(5):663–681.
21. Bijlsma L, Bade R, Been F, Celma A, Castiglioni S. Perspectives and challenges associated with the determination of new psychoactive substances in urine and wastewater: A tutorial. *Anal Chim Acta.* 2021 Feb 8;1145:132–147. doi:10.1016/j.aca.2020.08.058.
22. Gameli PS, Huestis MA, Balloni A, Busardò FP, Carlier J. Metabolism and detection of designer benzodiazepines: A systematic review. *Drug Metab Rev.* 2024 Nov;56(4):359–384. doi:10.1080/03602532.2024.2410747.
23. Klingberg J, Keen B, Cawley A, Pasin D, Fu S. Developments in high-resolution mass spectrometric analyses of new psychoactive substances. *Arch Toxicol.* 2022 Apr;96(4):949–967. doi: 10.1007/s00204-022-03224-2.
24. Prates Serrano JN, Benedito LE, de Souza MP, Maldaner AO, Oliveira AL. Quantitative NMR as a tool for analysis of new psychoactive substances. *Forensic Chem.* 2020;21:100282. doi: 10.1016/j.forc.2020.100282.
25. Graziano S, Anzillotti L, Mannocchi G, Pichini S, Busardò FP. Screening methods for rapid determination of new psychoactive substances (NPS) in conventional and non-conventional biological matrices. *J Pharm Biomed Anal.* 2019 Jan;163:170–179. doi:10.1016/j.jpba.2018.10.011.

26. Castaing-Cordier T, Ladroue V, Besacier F, et al. High-field and benchtop NMR spectroscopy for the characterization of new psychoactive substances. *Forensic Sci Int.* 2021 Apr;321:110718. doi:10.1016/j.forsciint.2021.110718.
27. Pasin D, Cawley A, Bidny S, Fu S. Current applications of high-resolution mass spectrometry for the analysis of new psychoactive substances: a critical review. *Anal Bioanal Chem.* 2017 Oct;409(25):5821–5836. doi:10.1007/s00216-017-0441-4.
28. Krajewski LC, Swanson KD, Bragg WA, et al. Application of the fentanyl analog screening kit toward the identification of emerging synthetic opioids in human plasma and urine by LC-QTOF. *Toxicol Lett.* 2020 Mar;320:87–94. doi:10.1016/j.toxlet.2019.12.007.
29. Oberacher H, Arnhard K. Compound identification in forensic toxicological analysis with untargeted LC-MS-based techniques. *Bioanalysis.* 2015 Nov;7(21):2825–2840. doi:10.4155/bio.15.193.
30. Salomone A, Di Corcia D, Negri P, et al. Targeted and untargeted detection of fentanyl analogues and their metabolites in hair by means of UHPLC-QTOF-HRMS. *Anal Bioanal Chem.* 2021 Jan;413(1):225–233. doi:10.1007/s00216-020-02994-x.
31. Niessen WM. Fragmentation of toxicologically relevant drugs in positive-ion liquid chromatography-tandem mass spectrometry. *Mass Spectrom Rev.* 2011 Jul–Aug;30(4):626–663. doi:10.1002/mas.20318.
32. Mardal M, Andreasen MF, Mollerup CB, et al. HighResNPS.com: An online crowd-sourced HR-MS database for suspect and non-targeted screening of new psychoactive substances. *J Anal Toxicol.* 2019 Aug 23;43(7):520–527. doi:10.1093/jat/bkz061.
33. Wang F, Pasin D, Skinnider MA, et al. Deep learning-enabled MS/MS spectrum prediction facilitates automated identification of novel psychoactive substances. *Anal Chem.* 2023 Dec 19;95(50):18326–18334. doi:10.1021/acs.analchem.3c02413.
34. Carlier J, Berardinelli D, Montanari E, Sirignano A, Di Trana A, Busardò FP. 3F-α-pyrrolydinovalerophenone (3F-α-PVP) in vitro human metabolism: Multiple in silico predictions to assist in LC-HRMS/MS analysis and targeted/untargeted data mining. *J Chromatogr B Analyt Technol Biomed Life Sci.* 2022 Mar 15;1193:828–837. doi: 10.1016/j.jchromb.2022.123162.
35. Wang M, Carver JJ, Phelan VV, et al. Sharing and community curation of mass spectrometry data with Global Natural Products Social Molecular Networking. *Nat Biotechnol.* 2016;34:828–837. doi:10.1038/nbt.3597.
36. Quinn RA, Nothias LF, Vining O, Meehan M, Esquenazi E, Dorrestein PC. Molecular networking as a drug discovery, drug metabolism, and precision medicine strategy. *Trends Pharmacol Sci.* 2017;38:143–154. doi:10.1016/j.tips.2016.10.011.
37. Yang JY, Sanchez LM, Rath CM, et al. Molecular networking as a dereplication strategy. *J Nat Prod.* 2013;76:1686–1699. doi:10.1021/np400413s.
38. Vincenti F, Montesano C, Di Ottavio F, et al. Molecular networking: A useful tool for the identification of new psychoactive substances in seizures by LC-HRMS. *Front Chem.* 2020 Nov;8:572952. doi: 10.3389/fchem.2020.572952.
39. Magny R, Lefrère B, Roulland E, et al. Feature-based molecular network for new psychoactive substance identification: The case of synthetic cannabinoids in a seized e-liquid and biological samples. *J Am Soc Mass Spectrom.* 2024 Oct 2;35(10):2276–2287. doi:10.1021/jasms.4c00009.
40. Banister SD, Wilkinson SM, Longworth M, et al. The synthesis and pharmacological evaluation of adamantane-derived indoles: Cannabimimetic drugs of abuse. *ACS Chem Neurosci.* 2013;4:1081–1092. doi:10.1021/cn400145h.
41. Kevin RC, Mirlohi S, Manning JJ, et al. Putative synthetic cannabinoids MEPIRAPIM, 5F-BEPIRAPIM (NNL-2), and their analogues are t-type calcium channel (CaV3) inhibitors. *ACS Chem Neurosci.* 2022;13:1395–1409. doi:10.1021/acschemneuro.1c00822.
42. Yasi EA, Kruyer NS, Peralta-Yahya P. Advances in G protein-coupled receptor high-throughput screening. *Curr Opin Biotechnol.* 2020 Aug;64:210–217. doi:10.1016/j.copbio.2020.06.004.

43. Mohd Fauzi F, Koutsoukas A, Cunningham A, Gallegos A, Sedefov R, Bender A. Computer-aided (in silico) approaches in the mode-of-action analysis and safety assessment of ostarine and 4-methylamphetamine. *Hum Psychopharmacol.* 2013;28:365–378. doi:10.1002/hup.2322.
44. Awale M, Reymond JL. Web-based tools for polypharmacology prediction. *Methods Mol. Biol.* 2019;1888:255–272. doi:10.1007/978-1-4939-8891-4_15.
45. Di Trana A, Brunetti P, Giorgetti R, et al. In silico prediction, LC-HRMS/MS analysis, and targeted/untargeted data-mining workflow for the profiling of phenylfentanyl in vitro metabolites. *Talanta* 2021;235:122740. doi:10.1016/j.talanta.2021.122740.
46. Gertsch J, Chicca A. CNS drug discovery in academia: Where basic research meets innovation. *Chembiochem.* 2024;25:e202400397. doi:10.1002/cbic.202400397.
47. Hanks JB, González-Maeso J. Animal models of serotonergic psychedelics. *ACS Chem Neurosci.* 2013 Jan 16;4(1):33–42. doi:10.1021/cn300138m.
48. Hunt PR. The *C. elegans* model in toxicity testing. *J Appl Toxicol.* 2017;37(1):50–59. doi:10.1002/jat.3357.
49. Engleman EA, Katner SN, Neal-Beliveau BS. *Caenorhabditis elegans* as a model to study the molecular and genetic mechanisms of drug addiction. *Prog Mol Biol Transl Sci.* 2016;137:229–252. doi:10.1016/bs.pmbts.2015.10.019.
50. Guha S, Calarco S, Gachet MS, Gertsch J. Juniperonic acid biosynthesis is essential in *Caenorhabditis elegans* lacking Δ6 desaturase (fat-3) and generates new ω-3 endocannabinoids. *Cells.* 2020 Sep 19;9(9):21–27. doi:10.3390/cells9092127.
51. Ide S, Ikeda K. *Caenorhabditis elegans* for opioid addiction research. *Curr Opin Neurobiol.* 2024;88:102914. doi:10.1016/j.conb.2024.102914.
52. Kautu BB, Phillips J, Steele K, Mengarelli MS, Nord EA. A behavioral survey of the effects of kavalactones on *Caenorhabditis elegans* neuromuscular transmission. *J Exper Neurosci.* 2017;11:1179069517705384. doi:10.1177/1179069517705384.
53. Freitas-Santos J, Brito IRR, Santana-Melo I, et al. Effects of cocaine, nicotine, and marijuana exposure in *Drosophila melanogaster* development: A systematic review and meta-analysis. *Prog Neuropsychopharmacol Biol Psychiatry.* 2024;134:111049.
54. Ferreira PMP, Ramos CLS, Filho JIAB, et al. Laboratory and physiological aspects of substitute metazoan models for in vivo pharmacotoxicological analysis. *Naunyn Schmiedebergs Arch Pharmacol.* 2024 Sep 19. doi:10.1007/s00210-024-03437-5.
55. Kawahara G, Maeda H, Kikura-Hanajiri R, Yoshida KI, Hayashi YK. The psychoactive drug 25B-NBOMe recapitulates rhabdomyolysis in zebrafish larvae. *Forens Toxicol.* 2017;35(2):369–375. doi:10.1007/s11419-017-0366-9.
56. Kirla KT, Groh KJ, Poetzsch M, et al. Importance of toxicokinetics to assess the utility of zebrafish larvae as a model for psychoactive drug screening using meta-chlorophenylpiperazine (mCPP) as an example. *Front Pharmacol.* 2018;9:414. doi:10.3389/fphar.2018.00414.
57. Pesavento S, Bilel S, Murari M, et al. Zebrafish larvae: A new model to study behavioral effects and metabolism of fentanyl, in comparison to a traditional mice model. *Med Sci Law.* 2022;62(3):188–198. doi:10.1177/00258024221074568.

4

Stimulant New Psychoactive Substances

Fabrizio Schifano, John Martin Corkery, Valeria Catalani, Stefania Chiappini, Davide Arillotta, Alessandro Vento, Norbert Scherbaum, and Amira Guirguis

4.1. Introduction

Apart from cocaine/crack cocaine, stimulants ("uppers") represent a diverse range of molecules that typically include psychedelic phenylethylamines, a variety of amphetamine-type stimulants (ATS), synthetic cathinones, some prescription drugs with abuse liability/potential, and a range of new/novel/emerging psychoactive substances (NPS) with mood/energy-enhancing properties.[1] There are several reasons for using "uppers," including: hallucinogenic experiences, euphoria, mood enhancement, increased self-confidence, openness in communication, empathy, mental clarity, increased alertness, insomnia, stimulation, intensification of sensory experiences, increased energy, reduced appetite, increased sociability, and increased libido and sexual performance.[2] Ease of access, possibly through web-based acquisition activities; perceived legality; assumed high purity; perceived better highs and safer to use compared to traditional stimulants; and short duration of action have all been cited as reasons for using stimulants.[3] Given the increasingly large number of stimulant NPS that have recently been identified,[4] we aim here to comment on the pharmacological, clinical pharmacological, toxicity, and treatment/management issues pertaining to a range of novel stimulants, including psychedelic phenethylamines; novel amphetamine-like molecules; synthetic cathinones; synthetic cocaine analogues; and methylphenidate-like novel psychoactive substances.

4.2. Methods

To identify those studies that are here deemed as representative, we searched Medline/PubMed since inception, and in all languages available, for studies using the terms "stimulants," "stimulant NPS," "new psychoactive substances," "novel psychoactive substances," "legal highs," "designer drugs," "research chemicals," "smart drugs," and "emerging drugs of abuse." A range of keyword strings (e.g., NPS AND medical consequences; psychopathological disturbances in novel stimulant users; etc.) were used. Both review and research (e.g., quantitative and qualitative) studies on NPS stimulant use have been included, while studies focusing on preclinical trials have been excluded from the review.

4.3. Popular Novel Stimulants

An overview of the different stimulant drugs is here offered, with a focus on: psychedelic phenethylamines; 2C-series molecules; aminoindanes; benzofurans; B-Fly; NBOMEs; ATS; 4-4'-DMAR; synthetic cathinones; MPH-like drugs; and synthetic cocaine analogues.

4.3.1. Psychedelic Phenethylamines

This group includes a large range of natural or synthetic substances that possess psychostimulant, entactogenic, and hallucinogenic effects, with mescaline representing the prototype psychoactive phenethylamine compound.[5] These molecules include TMA (3,4,5-trimethoxyamphetamine), DOM (3-methoxy-4,5-methylenedioxyamphetamine), DOET (2,4,4-trimethoxyamphetamine), DOI (4-iodo-2,5-dimethoxyamphetamine), and DOC (4-chloro-2,5-dimethoxyamphetamine), among others—all of which have consciousness-altering and sensory perception-distorting properties.[6] Alongside these substances, the group of phenethylamines also includes a large number of "classical" phenethylamines/MDMA (3,4-methylenedioxymethamphetamine)-like drugs (e.g., MDA [3,4-methylenedioxy- amphetamine]; MDEA [3,4-methylenedioxyethamphetamine]; MBDB [N-methyl-1-(1,3-benzodioxol-5-yl)-2-butanamine]; 2C- molecules; indanes; benzofurans; the latest generation of phenethylamine derivatives: e.g., "Bromo-dragonFLY"

(1-(8-bromobenzo[1,2-b; 4,5-b′]difuran-4-yl)-2-aminopropane); and NBOMe derivatives.[6]

4.3.2. 2C- Series Compounds

The MDMA-like 2C- molecules, such as 2C-B (Nexus, 2,5-dimethoxy-4-bromophenethylamine), 2C-I (2,5-dimethoxy-4-iodophenethylamine), 2C-E (2,5-dimethoxy-4-ethylphenethylamine), and 2C-D (2,5-dimethoxy-4-methylphenethylamine), are frequently ingested as MDMA substitutes and/or in association with other club drugs (e.g., MDMA, MBDB, ketamine, etc.). These compounds act primarily as agonists at the 5-HT_{2A} over 5-HT_{1A} receptors.[7] The 5-HT2A receptor stimulation is associated with the occurrence the hallucinogenic effects of these compounds.[8] Furthermore, most of the 2C- drugs also display low binding affinity to D_2 receptors and low inhibitory activity with monoamine transporters.[2,6]

4.3.3. Aminoindanes

The most popular aminoindanes, which are related to fenfluramine, include 5,6-methylenedioxy-2-aminoindane (MDAI; "MDAI gold"), 5-iodo-2-aminoindane, and 2-aminoindane (2-AI; "Pink Champagne"). Other aminoindanes, classified as stimulant NPS, include N-methyl-2AI, 1-aminoindane, and ETAI (N-ethyl-5-trifluoromethyl-2-aminoindane). The potential of aminoindanes to affect serotonin release and reuptake is likely to be associated with MDMA-like entactogenic and empathogenic effects.[9] Most aminoindanes are available from a variety of sources, including the internet, as powder, capsules, and tablets, and can be snorted or ingested. Aminoindanes users report hallucinogenic experiences, euphoria, mood enhancement, openness, empathy, mental clarity, stimulation, increased energy, and increased libido.[6,9]

4.3.4. Benzofurans

Benzofurans are phenethylamines structurally related to MDMA and MDA. Their chemical class includes several compounds, for example, 6-APB (6-[2-aminopropyl] benzofuran, or "BenzoFury"); 5-APB (s [5-(2-aminopropyl) benzofuran]); 6-APDB (6-[2-Aminopropyl]-2,3-dihydrobenzofuran, or "4-Desoxy-MDA"); 5-APDB (5-[2-Aminopropyl]-2,3-dihydrobenzofuran, or "3-Desoxy-MDA"); among others.[10,11] They are typically ingested orally since nasal insufflation may be painful. Their intake may be associated with stimulant, entactogenic, and hallucinogenic effects.[12]

4.3.5. Latest Generation Phenethylamine Derivatives; Bromo-DragonFLY

Bromo-dragonFLY (or "DOB-dragonfly"/"3C-Bromo-dragonfly") displays a high affinity for 5-HT_{2A}, 5-HT_{2B}, and 5-HT_{2C} receptors.[13] Long lasting (up to 72 hours) hallucinations, mood elevation, paranoid ideation, confusion, anxiety, and flashbacks have been described after its intake.[14]

4.3.6. Latest Generation Phenethylamine Derivatives; NBOMEs

Recently, several highly active N-benzyl substituted phenethylamines (NBOMEs) have become available, including 25B-NBOMe (2-(4-bromo-1,5-dimethoxyphenyl)-N-(2-methoxybenzyl) ethanamine), 25C-NBOMe (2-(4-chloro-2,5-dimethoxyphenyl)-N-[(2-methoxyphenyl) methyl] ethanamine, or "N-Bomb," "Pandora"), 25I-NBOMe (4-iodo-2,5-dimethoxy-N-(2-methoxybenzyl)phenethylamine, or "N-bomb," "Smiles," "CIMBI-5").[15] In vitro receptor studies have demonstrated that NBOMe compounds act as potent full agonists at the 5-HT_{2A} and 5-HT_{2C} receptors. Additionally, 25I-NBOMe and 25C-NBOMe are pharmacologically active at very low (sub-milligram) doses; and their higher affinity for the 2A receptor, compared to their 2C- derivatives, explain their higher incidence of hallucinations and delusions.[16] NBOMe-containing products are usually sold as tablets, capsules, powder, liquid, spray, and preloaded paper doses (blotters). They are usually taken orally (sublingually or buccally) or via nasal insufflations. Depending on the route of administration, their effects may last some 3–6 hours.[15] Psychotropic effects commonly reported may include euphoria, increased sociability, visual/auditory/olfactory/tactile sensations, hallucinations, life-changing spiritual experiences, empathy, psychedelic experiences, depersonalization, dissociation, and derealization.

4.3.7. Amphetamine-Type Substances (ATS)

Amphetamine-type substances include PMA (4-methoxyamphetamine, "Dr. Death"), PMMA (4-methoxymethamphetamine), 4-MTA (4-methylthioamphetamine, "flatliners"), DMA (2,5-dimethoxyamphetamine), and MPA (methiopropamine), among others.[17] From the pharmacodynamic point of view, PMA and PMMA ("Dr. Death") are similar to MDMA; however, both are more potent. Their ingestion may be associated with a fatal rise in body temperature, euphoria, a sense of full energy, an amplification of sounds/colors, and feelings of love/sociability. Methiopropamine acts as a selective NE/DA reuptake inhibitor.[18] It may be ingested, snorted, or smoked. At low doses, it is a stimulant associated with mild euphoria, alertness, sexual arousal, loss of appetite, tachycardia, and anxiety.[6]

4.3.8. Novel Psychostimulants; 4,4′-DMAR

A derivative of the anorectic aminorex, 4,4′-dimethylaminorex (4,4′-DMAR, "Serotoni") is a powerful dopamine/NE releaser and a serotonin transport inhibitor (SERT).[19] It may be snorted, or ingested, to achieve levels of both elation and increased alertness. The relating anxiety/agitation may be associated with an increase in body temperature and occurrence of cardiorespiratory problems. Clinical effects arise within 10–60 minutes and may last several hours.[6] Symptoms are mainly stimulant-like (i.e., euphoria, anorectic effect, alertness, etc.).

4.3.9. Synthetic Cathinones

Cathinones are synthetic analogues of naturally occurring phenethylamine alkaloids present in khat trees.[20] The most popular cathinone, mephedrone (4-ethylmethcathinone), was originally synthesized in 1929. By 2009, the popularity of cathinones worldwide was already vast, and the public health risk posed by these substances became evident. This resulted in the "first generation" cathinones ban,[21] which led to the emergence of a "second generation" of cathinones often referred to as "NRG." Generally NRG products included naphyrone, with those purchased over the internet showing the inclusion of other cathinones as well, such as mephedrone, flephedrone,

3,4-methylenedioxypyrovalerone (MDPV), butylone, and pentylone.[22] The popularity of cathinone use reached a climax in 2012 in Europe.

Recently, over 180 synthetic cathinones have been identified.[23] Of the cathinones notified to date to the European Monitoring Centre for Drugs and Drugs Addiction (EMCDDA), those of particular concern include mephedrone, 4-MEC/4-methylethcathinone, alpha-PVP/α-pyrrolidinopentiophenone, flephedrone, 3′,4′-methylenedioxy-α-pyrrolidinobutyrophenone (MDPBP), MDPV, methedrone, methylone, naphyrone, pentedrone, and pyrovalerone.

The "honeymoon" period for mephedrone lasted for a few years; users ceased their "love affair" with mephedrone, in part, due to its range of serious adverse effects, increased price, reduced availability or quality, and in part due to the increased availability and quality of amphetamines, cocaine, and ecstasy/MDMA.[24]

Cathinones have been classified on the basis of their pharmacological action (i.e., dopamine-DAT/serotonin-SERT/norepinephrine transporter-NET inhibition ratio) and comparability with traditional drugs of abuse, in particular:

1. *Cocaine/MDMA-mixed cathinones*, representing substrates for the DAT, SERT, and NET, including: mephedrone, 4-MEC, methylone, ethylone, butylone, and naphyrone; entactogenic, MDMA-like, effect when ingested orally, and with a psychostimulant cocaine-like effect when being administered intranasally.[25]
2. *Methamphetamine-like cathinones*, exhibiting high inhibitory potencies at DAT and lower inhibitory potencies at SERT,[26] while also inducing both DA and NE release similar to methamphetamine:[25] cathinone, methcathinone, flephedrone, ethcathinone, and 3-FMC.
3. *MDMA-like cathinones*, exhibiting a greater inhibitory potency at SERT compared to their inhibition at DAT, while inducing the release of both NE and 5-HT similar to the amphetamine analogues paramethoxymethamphetamine (PMA) and paramethoxyamphetamine (PMMA): 4-trifluoromethylmethcathinone and methedrone.[26]
4. *Pyrovalerone-cathinones*, exhibiting inhibitory potency at DAT and NET equal or greater than cocaine or methamphetamine and all readily crossing the blood–brain barrier (BBB) due to their high lipophilicity:[27] pyrovalerone, MDPV, and α-PVP. Due to these characteristics, these molecules may present with a high abuse potential.[2]

Synthetic cathinones are typically sold as pills, capsules, and powders. They are usually snorted/sniffed (insufflated), taken orally by "bombing" (swallowing the powder wrapped in a cigarette paper), mixed in a drink, or through intravenous injection.[28] Mephedrone possesses a re-dosing risk due to a half-life as short as 1 hour; in contrast, MDPV is thought to have a half-life of 3–5 hours.[29]

Synthetic cathinones are used for a variety of reasons, including euphoria, stimulation, increased energy, empathy, openness, mood enhancement, mental clarity, hallucinogenic experiences, and increased libido. Within the "chem sex" context, and especially so in the men who have sex with men (MSM) sub-population,[30] the intravenous synthetic cathinones/mephedrone misuse has been described in association with methamphetamine and/or gamma-hydroxybutyrate/gamma-butyrolactone (GHB/GBL). This scenario may include unprotected sex practice with an average of five sexual partners per session; sharing syringes; and highly elevated risk of the spread of blood-borne/sexually transmitted diseases.[30]

4.3.10. MPH-Like NPS

Methylphenidate (MPH) is a popular prescription drug worldwide that is being misused as a cognitive enhancer. However, any possible modification of cognitive performance may be related to drug-related improvements in subjective well-being.[31] Furthermore, a dose-response relationship, characterized by an inverted U-shaped curve (e.g., at higher doses, the more intense the effects, hence more detrimental for cognitive function), could occur.[32] Ethylphenidate (EPH; "Burst," "El Blanco," "Gogaine") is the MPH ethyl-homolog; both EPH and MPH are potent inhibitors of DA and NE reuptake, although EPH is almost 5 times less potent against NE than DA, and MPH is less selective.[33] Other popular MPH-derived compounds include 3,4-dichloromethylphenidate (3,4-DCMP), methylnaphthidate (HDMP-28), propylphenidate, and isopropylphenidate; 3,4-DCMP is claimed to be more potent than MPH, with a slower onset of action and longer duration.[33] HDMP-28 acts as a triple receptor reuptake inhibitor (DA, NE, and 5-HT) in a manner similar to cocaine; it is also claimed to have several times the potency of MPH, but with a shorter duration of action.[33] EPH can also be found as an additive ingredient in mixtures of psychoactive compounds, together with methiopropamine (MPA), ephedrine, phenylethylamine, and the remaining stimulants.[33,34] EPH intake can occur orally, intranasally, rectally, or through intramuscular/intravenous injection. The commonly reported dosages of EPH are 10–100 mg for oral or intranasal administration and 5–50 mg for injection.[35] The mean onset time for the "high" is around 15 minutes for intranasal administration and 25 minutes for oral administration; the mean duration of the effects is 120 minutes for all routes of administration. Common desired effects reported by users include euphoria, stimulation/increased arousal, improved concentration, sociability, and sexual drive.

4.3.11. Synthetic Cocaine Analogues

"Synthetic cocaine" is the slang term used for substances that are sold online as a legal alternative to cocaine.[36] Dimethocaine and 4-fluorotropacocaine (pFBT), typically found as white powder, act as DA reuptake inhibitors, resulting in mild stimulant effects. Similar to cocaine, both substances are being insufflated, because if consumed orally, they would be hydrolyzed by the digestive system esterases. Dimethocaine users report a short-lasting rush, together with increased levels of attention/concentration, talkativeness, and the desire to re-dose.[36] Further cocaine analogues include RTI-111 (dichloropane ((-)-2β-carbomethoxy-3β-(3,4-dichlorophenyl)tropane), a potent stimulant acting as an inhibitor of 5-HT, DA, and NE reuptake; RTI 121 ((-)-2β-carboisopropoxy-3β-(4-iodophenyl)tropane, RTI-121, IPCIT) and RTI-126 ((-)-2β-(1,2,4-oxadiazol-5-methyl)-3β-phenyltropane). RTI-121 is a potent/long-lasting stimulant acting as a selective DA reuptake inhibitor.[37] RTI-126, on the other hand, may present with a potency which is 5-fold higher than that of cocaine.[38] When snorted, these compounds are associated with alertness, euphoria, talkativeness, insomnia, prolonged residual tension/anxiety, and crash-like symptoms.[6]

4.4. NPS Stimulant-Related Acute Intoxication Signs/Symptoms and Fatalities Risk

An overview of the range of both signs and symptoms associated with the intake of stimulant NPS is here provided.

4.4.1. Psychedelic Phenethylamines

MDMA, together with related substances such as PMA and PMMA, may be associated with both severe serotonin syndrome and sympathomimetic effects.[36] It has been argued that common side effects, such as nystagmus, trismus, mild confusion, and hot flashes, are the low end of the serotonergic overactivity spectrum, which has at the higher end serotonin syndrome and death.[39] Typical side effects may be reported by more than half of a sample of users, and may include nausea/vomiting, headache, hallucinations, dizziness, palpitations, hyperthermia, seizures, agitation, abdominal cramps, jaw clenching, dry mouth, sweating, feeling cold and shivering, with a minority having experienced urinary retention and decreased libido.[39] Severe anxiety/panic or psychosis can be observed as well.[40]

Ecstasy can cause liver failure as a subacute effect that can emerge over the days after use. Patients may present in a critical condition, with liver encephalopathy, and some will require transplantation.[41] Pneumomediastinum and dilutional hyponatraemia/hyponatraemic encephalopathy may be a cause of ecstasy fatalities, particularly in women.[40] MDMA-related fatalities can follow sudden collapse and cardiac arrest or can result from disseminated intravascular coagulation, prolonged seizures, and multiple organ failure. Many of these result from extreme hyperthermia.[40]

Aminoindanes are reported to cause eye and skin irritation, as well as gastrointestinal disturbances with nausea, vomiting/diarrhea, and respiratory tract concerns. Three deaths associated with MDAI use, either alone or in combination, were identified in the United Kingdom during 2011–2012, all involving symptoms consistent with serotonin syndrome.[42] Intake of 2C- series compounds has been associated with headache, fever, dysphoria, sometimes hallucinations, mydriasis, seizures, severe agitation, and overall with serotonin syndrome.[43]

Several cases of acute intoxications and fatalities have been associated with Bromo-dragonFLY ingestion.[14]

NBOMes' untoward effects may include nausea, vomiting, headache, temporary dysuria, sweating, panic, severe agitation, aggressiveness, seizures, insomnia, and, sometimes, rhabdomyolysis with subsequent acidosis and renal failure, muscle rigidity, and cardiopulmonary arrest.[15] Several fatalities have been reported following the intake of NBOMe compounds.[44]

Benzofurans' adverse effects may include dry mouth, nausea, jaw/teeth clenching, insomnia, diarrhea, light hypersensitivity, hot flushes, headache, drowsiness, panic attacks/anxiety, depression, severe paranoia, and psychosis. An unpleasant "comedown," lasting several days, has been reported. Several deaths related to 5- and 6-APB have been identified.[11]

4.4.2. Amphetamine-Type Substances

An increasing number of fatalities have been described following PMA/PMMA consumption. The latter are particularly associated with severe and life-threatening symptoms, such as seizures and coma.[45] The untoward effects of 4,4′-DMAR include agitation, hyperthermia, breathing problems, cardiac arrest, and fatalities.[46]

4.4.3. Synthetic Cathinones

Synthetic cathinones display sympathomimetic effects (including tachycardia and hypertension, as well as psychoactive effects) similar to amphetamine derivatives. The Euro-DEN project compiled information on 10,709 emergency department (ED) admissions across 16 centers in 10 European cities for the period 2014–2015. NPS accounted for 7.3% of total ED admissions, of which 61.2% were cathinones, and mephedrone in 73.9% of these.[47] Conversely, in a retrospective study conducted in Germany over a 6-year period between January 2010 and January 2016, cathinones that were related to higher rates of intoxication were MDPV, methylone, and 3-MMC.[48]

Most frequent unwanted effects after the ingestion of synthetic cathinones would be as follows (in decreasing order): excessive sweating, headaches, palpitations, nausea, and cold blue fingers and toes. Similarly, in a Scottish student survey, more than half of those who had used mephedrone reported having at least one unwanted effect, with the following frequency: bruxism, paranoia, sore nasal passages, hot flushes, sore mouth/throat, nose bleeds, suppressed appetite, blurred vision, palpitations, insomnia, hallucinations, nausea/vomiting, and blue/cold extremities.[36]

Psychiatric unwanted side effects may indeed include aggression, combative behavior, confusion, extreme paranoia, delusions, hallucinations, paraesthesia, self-harm, and harm to others. Acute medical issues reported have included adverse cardiovascular effects, abdominal pain, chills, flushing, sweating, hyperthermia, renal failure, rhabdomyolysis, abnormalities of metabolic/blood tests such as elevated creatine kinase and hypokalaemia, and acidosis.[2]

A range of synthetic cathinones (including mephedrone, methylone, butylone, ethylone, a-PVP, MDPV, and methedrone) has been associated with fatalities.[2,28,29] A large number of fatalities related to cathinones may be associated with hangings and mechanical suicides.[49]

4.4.4. MPH-Like NPS

The adverse effects reported for MPH-like molecules include muscle tension, palpitations, sweating, appetite loss, anxiety/restlessness, insomnia, paranoia, and auditory/visual hallucinations.[50] EPH intake has been associated with bizarre/erratic and violent behavior, suicidality, psychosis, and clinical worsening of paranoid schizophrenia. A "crash"-like phase, after the end of an EPH binge session, with a period of mood lowering and fatigue, together with a strong urge/compulsion to re-dose and tolerance, has been described.[36] A range of fatalities associated with analytically confirmed EPH ingestion, mostly in combination with other drugs, have been described.[51]

4.4.5. Synthetic Cocaine Analogues

Related adverse/unwanted effects include peripheral vasoconstriction, tachycardia, diaphoresis, muscle twitching, nausea, and vomiting.[6]

4.5. NPS Stimulant-Related Chronic Intake and Long-Term Adverse Health Effects

An overview of the long-term adverse health effects of the vast range of stimulant NPS is here provided.

4.5.1. Amphetamine-Type Stimulants and Psychedelic Amphetamines

The main action of stimulants is on the cardiovascular system, due to their short- and long-term stimulation of the adrenergic system and consequent effects on blood pressure, cardiac modeling, atherogenesis, and cellular calcium signaling. Persistent psychostimulant use results in progressive cardiovascular pathology, largely in the form of accelerated atherosclerosis, hypertension, and myocardial ischaemia. Abstinence may result in some reversal of these issues.[1] Chronic use of ATS and related drugs has been associated with hepatocellular damage as well.[52]

Indeed, chronic ingestion of ATS-related drugs is typically associated with dependence, chronic depression, anxiety, sexual risk behavior, and increased risk of HIV and a tendency to suicide;[53] with chronic ATS ingestion, the occurrence of a drug-related psychosis has been widely described.[54]

Chronic use of ecstasy has been linked to serotonergic neurological damage and dysfunction, which some researchers have suggested may be responsible for a wide range of neuropsychiatric symptoms and cognitive impairments.[39] Significant trends indicating impairment may not typically be identified in those who have taken the drug on fewer than 50 occasions.[55] Users have described "mid-week blues" (e.g., fatigue, depressed mood, and decreased appetite) appearing 3–5 days after the use of ecstasy and likely to be associated with depleted serotonin.[56] A serotonergic valvular heart disease has also been associated with MDMA chronic use.[57] Chronic use of a mixture containing MDAI and 2-AI (the latter of which appears to be more amphetamine-like than MDMA-like) has been associated with one case of cyanosis caused by methemoglobinemia.[58]

4.5.2. Synthetic Cathinones

Synthetic cathinones present with a dependence potential, in being possibly "as or more addictive" than cocaine.[36] Tolerance to mephedrone develops rapidly, with users consuming higher doses more frequently; the development of cravings for mephedrone may be related to an increased frequency of use.[50] Unpleasant physical and mental symptoms may be experienced when going through withdrawal from mephedrone, methcathinone, and MDPV. Depression, anxiety, tiredness, insomnia, nasal congestion, and impaired concentration have been described as symptoms indicating mephedrone withdrawal.[59] Furthermore, α-PVP appears to cause extreme craving and risk of binge consumption.[60] Interestingly, a neonatal withdrawal syndrome was described in a baby whose mother was a chronic 4-MEC user; the newborn presented with increased jitteriness and irritability, high-pitched cry, hypertonia in the limbs, and brisk tendon reflexes.[61] Paranoid ideation and mood disturbances have been observed in chronic users of synthetic cathinones.[24,40] Finally, within the chem sex scenario, cathinones may frequently be present in association with both hepatitis C and HIV.[62]

4.6. Acute Stimulant NPS-Related Treatment and Management Options

The constantly and rapidly evolving NPS drug scenario represents a challenge for medicine, and especially so for both emergency physicians and mental health professionals.[4] The unknown composition of NPS mixtures represents a great challenge to the prediction of extent of toxicity and possibly resulting in a plethora of medical and psychopathological consequences.[6] One could argue that it is problematic to draft a good-for-all stimulant NPS treatment/management plan to cope with the behavioral and psychopathological disturbances related to the intake of the virtually hundreds of molecules currently available. Difficulties in ascribing effects to a specific drug/class of drug in the context of polysubstance use, especially where NPS use is known or suspected, may mean that the clinician is generally advised to treat the symptoms with which patients present.[28]

4.6.1. Medical Disturbances Optimal Treatment/Management Approach

In the acute setting, clinicians are unlikely to have the option of identifying known, let alone unknown, stimulant NPS in a timely manner. In fact, consumers of these molecules may present to the ED without providing information on the substances(s) ingested, and it is likely that standard drug tests will show negative results.[42] For patients presenting acute medical complications from NPS stimulant use, laboratory tests should include standardized urine drug tests, which can be helpful in identifying a possible concomitant intake of classic illicit substances, a complete blood cell count, a complete metabolic panel, electrocardiogram (ECG) baseline, and cardiac enzymes. Creatine phosphokinase is helpful if rhabdomyolysis is suspected on the basis of severe muscle spasms, swelling and pain in the extremities, or severe seizures.[23]

No specific antidotes are available for most NPS, apart from benzodiazepine and opioid antagonist compounds (e.g., respectively, flumazenil and naloxone). In case of cathinones intoxication with sympathomimetic complications and agitation, the use of benzodiazepine agonists seems appropriate.[63] The intake of serotonergic drugs (e.g., phenethylamines, hallucinogens, NBOMe compounds, etc.) may be associated with the occurrence of serotonin syndrome. Related hyperthermia must be evaluated and treated aggressively, which typically involves cooling measures, and intravenous fluid administration and hemodiafiltration could be used to filter myoglobin in the case of rhabdomyolysis.[64] Appropriate sedation paralysis and assisted ventilation may at times be needed. The serotonin syndrome is managed using benzodiazepines and cyproheptadine, although inpatient admission, possibly to intensive care units, may at times be needed.[63]

4.6.2. Psychopathological Disturbances Optimal Treatment/Management Approach

Indeed, stimulant NPS intake is typically associated with (a) increased central dopamine levels, mostly associated with novel psychedelic phenethylamines, synthetic cathinones, MPH-like NPS, cocaine analogues, and 4,4′-DMAR; and/or (b) intense 5-HT2A receptor activation, reported with both some cathinones and NBOMe compounds.[6] Therefore, a variety of related psychopathological disturbances can be observed.[36]

Placing the patient in a quiet, dark environment can be helpful. In case of agitation, the initial management of agitated patients should focus on decreasing levels of both self- and outward-directed aggression and agitation. Verbal de-escalation can always be considered with more cooperative patients.[2,28] When a medication is needed, given the complex/unknown pharmacology of the psychotropic substances arguably ingested, benzodiazepines, either intramuscular (IM) or intranasal midazolam, because of its fast absorption/onset of action, or lorazepam may be considered.[6] These molecules may be particularly useful for the treatment of stimulant/synthesized cathinone-related agitation and for stopping seizures.[64] Benzodiazepines, however, need frequent re-dosing/high dosages to achieve adequate sedative effects, and this may be a problem if clients have co-ingested alcohol.[2] Where patients cannot be controlled with benzodiazepines alone, propofol, dexmedetomidine, barbiturates, and/or antipsychotics may be considered, although this may further contribute to the acute toxicity effects of the abused substances.[6,65]

Drugs such as haloperidol, olanzapine, or ziprasidone can lower seizure thresholds, limit heat-dissipation levels, and contribute to dysrhythmias. People with underlying cardiac, neurological, and psychiatric conditions, especially those on medication, are likely to be at greatest risk of serious adverse events.[26]

Sympathomimetic and psychotic signs and symptoms of stimulant- (and NPS in general) related intoxication may significantly improve/resolve after 3–4 days.[64] From a more general point of view, in treating substance-induced psychotic disorders, second-generation antipsychotics (SGAs) may present with some advantages over first-generation ones, being the SGAs less frequently associated with interference at the drug-reward system level, hence not increasing levels of craving.[66] Furthermore, SGAs act as antagonists of the serotonin $5HT_{2A}$ receptor, the main target of most hallucinogenic drugs.[67]

4.7. Discussion and Conclusions

An updated narrative overview of the pharmacological, clinical pharmacological, toxicity, and treatment/management issues related to a variety of novel stimulants has been provided here. One of the main issues that emerged was related to the possible occurrence of intense, acute and chronic, medical, and psychopathological consequences related to the ingestion of stimulant NPS.

As with other stimulants, the treatment of harmful stimulant NPS use may need to include a psychosocial approach.[28] In most cases, users would be polydrug users, and existing interventions would be unlikely to focus on a single molecule in isolation. For stimulant users, a 45–60-minute clinical intervention/structured motivational discussion may need to include exploration of the individual's characteristics of use, desired and unwanted effects of stimulant NPS ingestion, and plans for behavioral changes.[36]

Given the serious health harms associated with novel stimulant ingestion, one would wonder about the best approach to convince clients to stop ingesting these molecules altogether. For the treatment of withdrawal/cravings, and although no specific "ad hoc" medications have been approved, the dopaminergic drug bupropion may represent an option.[28] Indeed, spontaneous reasons for discontinuing use can include both peer and social pressures, with negative consequences on relationships with family and friends possibly acting as an incentive to change.[36]

In comparison with well-known scheduled substances such as THC, cocaine, and heroin, there may be current relatively low levels of stimulant NPS use. However, the online market of NPS is unfortunately developing far more rapidly than academic research; in fact, a range of novel molecules are consistently offered to vulnerable customers not only through the most popular "open web" search engines, but also through the "deep web" and especially through its most hidden portion (i.e., the "dark net").[68] Current research activities, coordinated by our group and carried out with the help of an "ad hoc" web crawler navigating on a large range of psychonauts' websites, specialized fora, have identified an excess of 4300 NPS; out of these, some 1600 were stimulant NPS such as those described here.[43] Therefore, it could be argued that raising awareness and education of healthcare professionals about NPS health harms, interventions, harm-reduction techniques, and referral pathways are of paramount importance.

Indeed, future studies will provide better levels of NPS clinical and basic pharmacology-related knowledge, so that better tailored management/treatment guidelines can be made available. Health professionals' education involving knowledge on stimulant NPS health harms, potential interventions, and referral pathways is lacking. Future NPS-related tutoring activities will allow clinicians to promote health-prevention and educational activities, which in turn would reduce the negative social impact of NPS misuse, unnecessary hospital admissions, and avoidable fatalities.

References

1. Duflou J. Psychostimulant use disorder and the heart. *Addiction.* 2020;115(1):175–183. doi:10.1111/ADD.14713.
2. Schifano F, Papanti GD, Orsolini L, Corkery JM. Novel psychoactive substances: the pharmacology of stimulants and hallucinogens. *Expert Rev Clin Pharmacol.* 2016 Jul;9(7):943–954. doi:10.1586/17512433.2016.1167597.
3. Sutherland R, Bruno R, Peacock A, et al. Motivations for new psychoactive substance use among regular psychostimulant users in Australia. *Int J Drug Policy.* 2017;43:23–32. doi:10.1016/J.DRUGPO.2016.12.021.
4. Schifano F, Napoletano F, Chiappini S, et al. New/emerging psychoactive substances and associated psychopathological consequences. *Psychol Med.* 2021;51(1):30–42. doi:10.1017/S0033291719001727.
5. McLaughlin JL. Peyote: An introduction. *Lloydia* 1973;36(1):1–8. https://eurekamag.com/research/000/159/000159325.php. Accessed December 22, 2021.

6. Schifano F, Orsolini L, Duccio Papanti G, et al. Novel psychoactive substances of interest for psychiatry. *World Psychiatry*. 2015;14(1): 15–26. doi:10.1002/wps.20174.
7. Rickli A, Luethi D, Reinisch J, et al. Receptor interaction profiles of novel N-2-methoxybenzyl (NBOMe) derivatives of 2,5-dimethoxy-substituted phenethylamines (2C drugs). *Neuropharmacology*. 2015;99:546–553. doi:10.1016/j.neuropharm.2015.08.034.
8. Halberstadt AL, Geyer MA. Multiple receptors contribute to the behavioral effects of indoleamine hallucinogens. *Neuropharmacology*. 2011 Sep;61(3):364–381. doi:10.1016/j.neuropharm.2011.01.017. Epub 2011 Jan 20. PMID: 21256140.
9. Pinterova N, Horsley RR, Palenicek T. Synthetic aminoindanes: A summary of existing knowledge. *Front Psychiatry*. 2017;8:17. doi:10.3389/FPSYT.2017.00236.
10. King LA. New phenethylamines in Europe. *Drug Test Anal.* 2014;6(7–8):808–818. doi:10.1002/dta.1570.
11. Roque Bravo R, Carmo H, Carvalho F, et al. Benzo fury: A new trend in the drug misuse scene. *J Appl Toxicol.* 2019;39(8):1083–1095. doi:10.1002/JAT.3774.
12. Rickli A, Kopf S, Hoener MC, et al. Pharmacological profile of novel psychoactive benzofurans. *Br J Pharmacol.* 2015;172(13):3412–3425. doi:10.1111/bph.13128.
13. O'Connor RE, Keating JJ. Characterization of synthetic routes to "Bromo-DragonFLY" and benzodifuranyl isopropylamine homologues utilizing ketone intermediates. Part 1: Synthesis of ketone precursors. *Drug Test Anal.* 2014;6(7–8):658–667. doi:10.1002/DTA.1504.
14. Corazza O, Schifano F, Farre M, et al. Designer drugs on the internet: A phenomenon out-of-control? The emergence of hallucinogenic drug Bromo-Dragonfly. Curr Clin Pharmacol. 2011;6(2):125–129. doi:10.2174/157488411796151129.
15. Bersani FS, Corazza O, Albano G, Valeriani G, Santacroce R, Bolzan Mariotti Posocco F, Cinosi E, Simonato P, Martinotti G, Bersani G, Schifano F. 25C-NBOMe: preliminary data on pharmacology, psychoactive effects, and toxicity of a new potent and dangerous hallucinogenic drug. *Biomed Res Int.* 2014;2014:734749. doi:10.1155/2014/734749.
16. Srisuma S, Bronstein AC, Hoyte CO. NBOMe and 2C substitute phenylethylamine exposures reported to the National Poison Data System. *Clin Toxicol (Phila).* 2015;53(7):624–628. doi:10.3109/15563650.2015.1054502.
17. Kim JY, Suh S, Park J, et al. Simultaneous determination of amphetamine-related new psychoactive substances in urine by gas chromatography-mass spectrometry. *J Anal Toxicol.* 2018;42(9):605–616. doi:10.1093/JAT/BKY037.
18. Nguyen PT, Dang DK, Tran HQ, et al. Methiopropamine, a methamphetamine analogue, produces neurotoxicity via dopamine receptors. Chem-Biol Interact. 2019;305:134–147. doi:10.1016/J.CBI.2019.03.017.
19. Brandt SD, Baumann MH, Partilla JS, et al. Characterization of a novel and potentially lethal designer drug, (±)-cis-para-methyl-4-methylaminorex (4,4'-DMAR, or "Serotoni"). Drug Test Anal. 2014;6(0):684. doi:10.1002/DTA.1668.
20. Corkery JM. Khat-chewing it over: Continuing "cultural cement," cardiac challenge, or catalyst for change? In: Davies S, Johnston A, Holt D, eds. *Forensic Toxicology: Drug Use and Misuse.* Royal Society of Chemistry; 2016:165–207. https://books.google.it/books?hl=en&lr=&id=YkCuDAAAQBAJ&oi=fnd&pg=PA165&dq=Catha+edulis%3B+Corkery,+2016&ots=vqZtzQ6OcW&sig=IsvB6LOQzdG7P9wQ0yFZD0oFqg4#v=onepage&q=Catha edulis%3B Corkery%2C 2016&f=false. Accessed December 22, 2021.
21. Advisory Council on the Misuse of Drugs. ACMD report on the consideration of the cathinones. Available from: https://www.gov.uk/government/publications/acmd-report-on-the-consideration-of-the-cathinones?utm_source=chatgpt.com. Accessed December 8, 2025.
22. Valente MJ, Guedes De Pinho P, De Lourdes Bastos M, et al. Khat and synthetic cathinones: A review. *Arch Toxicol.* 2014; 88(1):15–45. doi:10.1007/S00204-013-1163-9.

23. Schifano F, Napoletano F, Arillotta D, et al. The clinical challenges of synthetic cathinones. *Br J Clin Pharmacol.* 2020;86(3):410–419. doi:10.1111/bcp.14132.
24. Guirguis A, Corkery JM, Stair JL, et al. Intended and unintended use of cathinone mixtures. *Human Psychopharmacol.* 2017;32(3). doi:10.1002/hup.2598.
25. Liechti ME. Novel psychoactive substances (designer drugs): Overview and pharmacology of modulators of monoamine signaling. Swiss Med Weekly. 2015;145:w14043. doi:10.4414/SMW.2015.14043.
26. Simmler LD, Rickli A, Hoener MC, et al. Monoamine transporter and receptor interaction profiles of a new series of designer cathinones. *Neuropharmacology.* 2014;79:152–160. doi:10.1016/J.NEUROPHARM.2013.11.008.
27. Simmler LD, Buser TA, Donzelli M, et al. Pharmacological characterization of designer cathinones in vitro. *Br J Pharmacol.* 2013;168(2):458. doi:10.1111/J.1476-5381.2012.02145.X.
28. Schifano F, Orsolini L, Papanti D, et al. NPS: Medical consequences associated with their intake. In: Baumann MH, Glennon RA, Wiley JL, eds. *Current Topics in Behavioral Neurosciences.* Springer Verlag; 2017:351–380. doi:10.1007/7854_2016_15.
29. Schifano F, Albanese A, Fergus S, et al. Mephedrone (4-methylmethcathinone; "meow meow"): Chemical, pharmacological and clinical issues. *Psychopharmacology (Berl).* 2011;214(3):593–602. doi:10.1007/S00213-010-2070-X.
30. Giorgetti R, Tagliabracci A, Schifano F, et al. When "chems" meet sex: A rising phenomenon called "chemsex." Curr Neuropharmacol. 2017;15(5):762. doi:10.2174/1570159x15666161117151148.
31. Batistela S, Bueno O, Vaz L, et al. Methylphenidate as a cognitive enhancer in healthy young people. *Dement Neuropsychol.* 2016;10(2):134–142. doi:10.1590/S1980-5764-2016DN1002009.
32. Linssen A, Sambeth A, Vuurman E, et al. Cognitive effects of methylphenidate in healthy volunteers: A review of single dose studies. *Int J Neuropsychopharmacol.* 2014;17(6):961–977. doi:10.1017/S1461145713001594.
33. ACMD. *Methylphenidate-Based NPS: A Review of the Evidence of Use and Harm.* The British Library; 2015. https://www.bl.uk/collection-items/methylphenidatebased-nps-a-review-of-the-evidence-of-use-and-harm. Accessed December 22, 2021.
34. WEDINOS. WEDINOS: Welsh Emerging Drugs & Identification of Novel Substances Project. 2021. https://www.wedinos.org/. Accessed December 22, 2021.
35. TripSit. TripSit factsheets: Ethylphenidate. 2021. https://drugs.tripsit.me/ethylphenidate. Accessed December 22, 2021.
36. Gannon BM, Baumann MH, Walther D, Jimenez-Morigosa C, Sulima A, Rice KC, Collins GT. The abuse-related effects of pyrrolidine-containing cathinones are related to their potency and selectivity to inhibit the dopamine transporter. *Neuropsychopharmacology.* 2018 Nov;43(12):2399–2407. doi:10.1038/s41386-018-0209-3.
37. Fleckenstein AE, Kopajtic TA, Boja JW, et al. Highly potent cocaine analogs cause long-lasting increases in locomotor activity. *Eur J Pharmacol.* 1996;311(2–3):109–114. doi:10.1016/0014-2999(96)00423-2.
38. Carroll FI, Blough BE, Nie Z, et al. Synthesis and monoamine transporter binding properties of 3β-(3′,4′-disubstituted phenyl)tropane-2β-carboxylic acid methyl esters. *J Med Chem.* 2005;48(8):2767–2771. doi:10.1021/JM040185A/SUPPL_FILE/JM040185A_S.PDF.
39. Parrott AC. Recreational ecstasy/MDMA, the serotonin syndrome, and serotonergic neurotoxicity. *Pharmacol Biochem Behav.* 2002;71(4):837–844. doi:10.1016/S0091-3057(01)00711-0.
40. Schifano F. A bitter pill: Overview of ecstasy (MDMA, MDA) related fatalities. *Psychopharmacology (Berl).* 2004;173(3–4):242–248. doi:10.1007/S00213-003-1730-5.

41. Cajanding RJM. MDMA-associated liver toxicity: Pathophysiology, management, and current state of knowledge. *AACN Adv Crit Care.* 2019;30(3):232–248. doi:10.4037/AACNACC2019852.
42. Corkery JM, Elliott S, Schifano F, et al. MDAI (5,6-methylenedioxy-2-aminoindane; 6,7-dihydro-5H-cyclopenta[f][1,3]benzodioxol-6-amine; "sparkle"; "mindy") toxicity: A brief overview and update. *Hum Psychopharmacol.* 2013;28(4):345–355. doi:10.1002/HUP.2298.
43. Schifano F, Chiappini S, Miuli A, et al. New psychoactive substances (NPS) and serotonin syndrome onset: A systematic review. *Exper Neurol.* 2021;339:113638. doi:10.1016/j.expneurol.2021.113638.
44. Kueppers VB, Cooke CT. 25I-NBOMe related death in Australia: A case report. *Forensic Sci Int.* 2015;249:e15–e18. doi:10.1016/j.forsciint.2015.02.010.
45. Yang C-A, Liu H-C, Liu RH, et al. Simultaneous quantitation of seven phenethylamine-type drugs in forensic blood and urine samples by UHPLC–MS-MS. *J Anal Toxicol.* 2022;46(3):246–256. doi:10.1093/JAT/BKAB014.
46. Loi B, Zloh M, De Luca MA, et al. 4,4′-Dimethylaminorex ("4,4′-DMAR"; "Serotoni") misuse: A web-based study. *Hum Psychopharmacol.* 2017;32(3):e2575. doi:10.1002/hup.2575.
47. Dines AM, Wood DM, Yates C, et al. Acute recreational drug and new psychoactive substance toxicity in Europe: 12 months data collection from the European Drug Emergencies Network (Euro-DEN). *Clin Toxicol (Phila).* 2015;53(9):893–900. doi:10.3109/15563650.2015.1088157.
48. Romanek K, Stenzel J, Schmoll S, et al. Synthetic cathinones in Southern Germany: Characteristics of users, substance-patterns, co-ingestions, and complications. *Clin Toxicol (Phila).* 2017;55(6):573–578. doi:10.1080/15563650.2017.1301463.
49. Chiappini S, Mosca A, Miuli A, et al. New psychoactive substances and suicidality: A systematic review of the current literature. *Medicina.* 2021;57(6):580. doi:10.3390/MEDICINA57060580.
50. Chen X, Faviez C, Schuck S, et al. Mining patients' narratives in social media for pharmacovigilance: adverse effects and misuse of methylphenidate. *Front Pharmacol.* 2018;9:541. doi:10.3389/FPHAR.2018.00541.
51. Maskell PD, Smith PR, Cole R, et al. Seven fatalities associated with ethylphenidate. *Forensic Sci Int.* 2016;265:70–74. doi:10.1016/J.FORSCIINT.2015.12.045.
52. Luethi D, Walter M, Zhou X, et al. Para-halogenation affects monoamine transporter inhibition properties and hepatocellular toxicity of amphetamines and methcathinones. Front Pharmacol. 2019;10(Apr):438. doi:10.3389/FPHAR.2019.00438/BIBTEX.
53. Armoon B, SoleimanvandiAzar N, Fleury MJ, et al. Prevalence, sociodemographic variables, mental health condition, and type of drug use associated with suicide behaviors among people with substance use disorders: A systematic review and meta-analysis. *J Addict Dis.* 2021;39(4):550–569. doi:10.1080/10550887.2021.1912572.
54. Huber M, Kirchler E, Karner M, et al. Delusional parasitosis and the dopamine transporter. A new insight of etiology? *Med Hypotheses.* 2007;68(6):1351–1358. doi:10.1016/J.MEHY.2006.07.061.
55. Schifano F. Potential human neurotoxicity of MDMA ("Ecstasy"): Subjective self-reports, evidence from an Italian drug addiction centre and clinical case studies. *Neuropsychobiology.* 2000;42(1):25–33. doi:10.1159/000026667.
56. Curran HV, Travill RA. Mood and cognitive effects of +/-3,4-methylenedioxymethamphetamine (MDMA, "ecstasy"): week-end "high"? followed by mid-week low. *Addiction.* 1997;92(7):821–831. doi:10.1111/J.1360-0443.1997.TB02951.X.
57. Bhattacharyya S, Schapira AH, Mikhailidis DP, et al. Drug-induced fibrotic valvular heart disease. *Lancet.* 2009;374(9689):577–585. doi:10.1016/S0140-6736(09)60252-X.

58. Green D, Barry P, Green HD. Central cyanosis on a psychiatric unit treated at the Salford Royal Hospital. *Thorax.* 2014;69(12):1157–1158. doi:10.1136/THORAXJNL-2014-205769.
59. Winstock AR, Mitcheson LR, Deluca P, et al. Mephedrone, new kid for the chop? *Addiction.* 2011;106(1):154–161. doi:10.1111/J.1360-0443.2010.03130.X.
60. Patocka J, Zhao B, Wu W, et al. Flakka: New dangerous synthetic cathinone on the drug scene. *Int J Mol Sci.* 2020;21(21):1–14. doi:10.3390/IJMS21218185.
61. Pichini S, Rotolo MC, García J, et al. Neonatal withdrawal syndrome after chronic maternal consumption of 4-methylethcathinone. *Forensic Sci Int.* 2014;245:e33–e35. doi:10.1016/J.FORSCIINT.2014.10.027.
62. Batisse A, Eiden C, Deheul S, et al. Chemsex practice in France: An update in Addictovigilance data. Fundam Clin Pharmacol. 2022;36(2):397–404. doi:10.1111/FCP.12725.
63. Schifano F, Chiappini S, Catalani V, et al. Psychobiological, medical, and psychiatric implications of new/novel psychoactive substance (NPS) use. In: *Psychobiological Issues in Substance Use and Misuse.* Routledge; 2020:213–233. doi:10.4324/9780429296345-11.
64. Corkery JM, Orsolini L, Papanti D, et al. Novel psychoactive substances (NPS) and recent scenarios: Epidemiological, anthropological and clinical pharmacological issues. *Comprehensive Series in Photochemical and Photobiological Sciences* 17. Royal Society of Chemistry; 2018:207–255. doi:10.1039/9781788010344-00207.
65. Kersten BP, McLaughlin ME. Toxicology and management of novel psychoactive drugs. *J Pharm Pract.* 2015;28(1):50–65. doi:10.1177/0897190014544814.
66. Juckel G. Inhibition of the reward system by antipsychotic treatment. *Dialogues Clin Neurosci.* 2016;18(1):109. doi:10.31887/DCNS.2016.18.1/GJUCKEL.
67. Valeriani G, Corazza O, Bersani FS, et al. Olanzapine as the ideal "trip terminator"? Analysis of online reports relating to antipsychotics' use and misuse following occurrence of novel psychoactive substance-related psychotic symptoms. *Hum Psychopharmacol.* 2015;30(4):249–254. doi:10.1002/HUP.2431.
68. Orsolini L, Papanti D, Corkery J, et al. An insight into the deep web: Why it matters for addiction psychiatry? *Hum Psychopharmacol.* 2017;32(3). doi:10.1002/hup.2573.

5

Synthetic Cannabinoid Receptor Agonists (SCRAs)

Philippe Pfeifer and Katharina Elisabeth Grafinger

5.1. Commonly Used Synthetic Cannabinoid Receptor Agonists (SCRAs)

5.1.1. History of SCRAs

There are 4 different classes of cannabinoids: phytocannabinoids (naturally occurring in plants), endocannabinoids (occurring in vivo), semi-synthetic cannabinoids (SSCs) (extracted from plant material) and synthetic cannabinoids (SCs) (chemically synthesized) (see Figure 5.1). SCs, also referred to as synthetic cannabinoid receptor agonists (SCRAs), include more than 270 monitored compounds, one of the biggest classes of new psychoactive substances (NPS).[1]

Originally starting in the 1980s,[2] SCRAs were developed and investigated for biomedical research purposes (e.g., to study their interaction with CB_1 and CB_2 receptors or to selectively activate the CB receptors)[3] and overall as potential therapeutic agents.[4] CB_1 agonists are investigated for a multitude of effects, such as multiple sclerosis (muscle relaxation), pain (analgesia), cancer (antiemetic and appetite-stimulating effect during chemotherapy), and glaucoma (lowering intraocular pressure).[5] Selective CB_2 agonists may have a potential application as anti-inflammatory analgesics without leading to cannabis-like intoxications (see section 4.2 on intoxications).[5] The first SCRAs sold in herbal blends as so-called "Spice" were the indolyl naphthyl ketone JWH-018 and the phenylcyclohexanol derivative CP-47,497 in December 2008.[6] Herbal blends (leaves laced with an SCRA) were the first form of distribution of SCRAs. Today they are also available as bulk

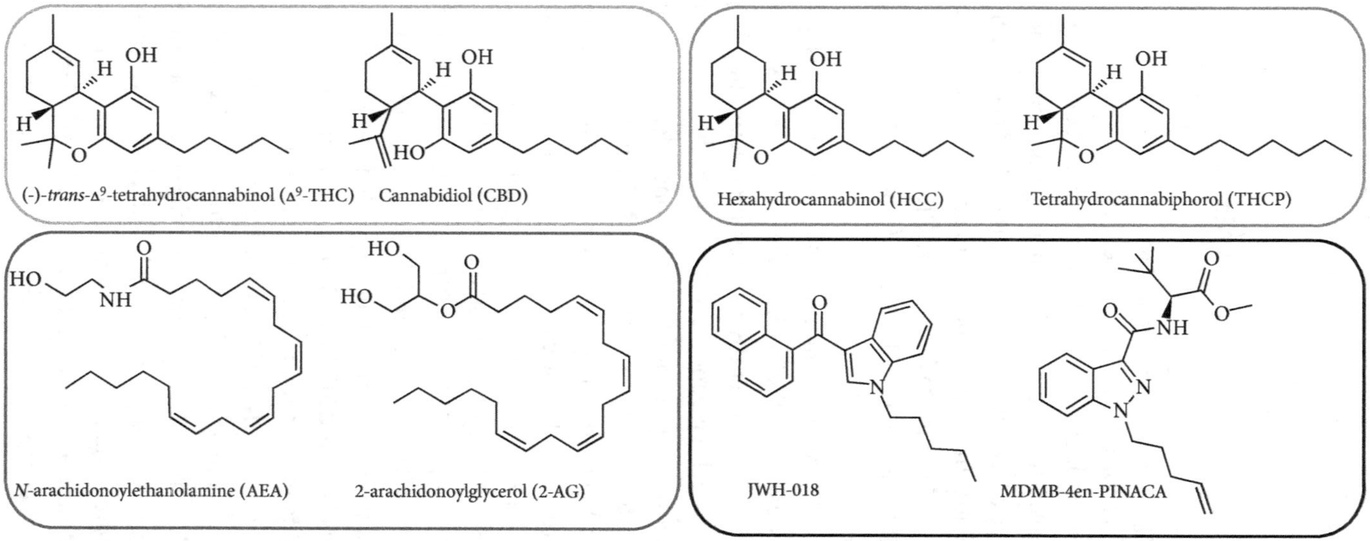

Figure 5.1. Chemical structures of examples of phytocannabinoids, semi-synthetic cannabinoids, endocannabinoids, and synthetic cannabinoids.

powders, tablets,[7] soaked or sprayed onto paper or textiles (for smuggling into prison),[8] e-liquids, or recently as waxy or putty-like materials.[9]

5.1.2. The SCRA Market

In the World Drug Report 2024, the United Nations Office on Drugs and Crime (UNODC) reported that 566 different NPS were on the drug market during that study period. Of those, SCRAs were the second-largest NPS class with 96 compounds. Moreover, the UNODC hypothesized, on the limited data available, that currently SCRAs were the NPS class with the largest prevalence worldwide. In 2022, in the European Union, 13% of all reported police seizures (i.e., 4543 cases) were due to SCRA intoxication. The vast majority of these SCRA seizures were herbal material (3056 cases, 233.5 kg) and powders (385 cases, 504 kg).[10]

The SCRA market is highly dynamic, with compounds disappearing and emerging continuously (see Figure 5.2). The first SCRAs were structurally very similar to Δ^9-THC. Currently, as a result of designing drugs strategically to circumvent legal regulations, SCRAs are highly structurally diverse. The European Union Drug Agency (EUDA) concludes that drug producers use national and international scheduling of NPS as an exclusion template for their range of offered products.[11] In this regard, it has been reported that novel legally controlled SCRAs are immediately removed from the NPS online drug market and are replaced by a new legal analogue.[12]

For 2022, the EUDA reported that the main SCRAs seized in Europe were ADB-BUTINCA, MDMB-4en-PINACA, Cumyl-NBMINACA, 4F-MDMB-BICA, 5F-MDMB-PICA, and JWH-210 (ordered in decreasing number of SCRAs seized as herbal material).[10] In powdered form, additionally ADB-B-5Br-INACA and 5F-AKB48 were the main seized compounds.

Until 2021, China was the main SCRA or SCRA-precursor manufacturer worldwide. However, in July 2021, China transitioned from a substance-specific regulatory framework, which controlled individual compounds (enumerated in the annexes of the law), to a class-wide ban on SCRAs, defined based on 7 core structural categories.[13] This class-wide ban included the indole/indazole core structures, which were prominent on the NPS market until 2021. At that time, ADB-BUTINACA and MDMB-4en-PINACA were the most prominent compounds on the NPS market; however, due to their indazole core, they were both legally controlled after the class-wide ban.

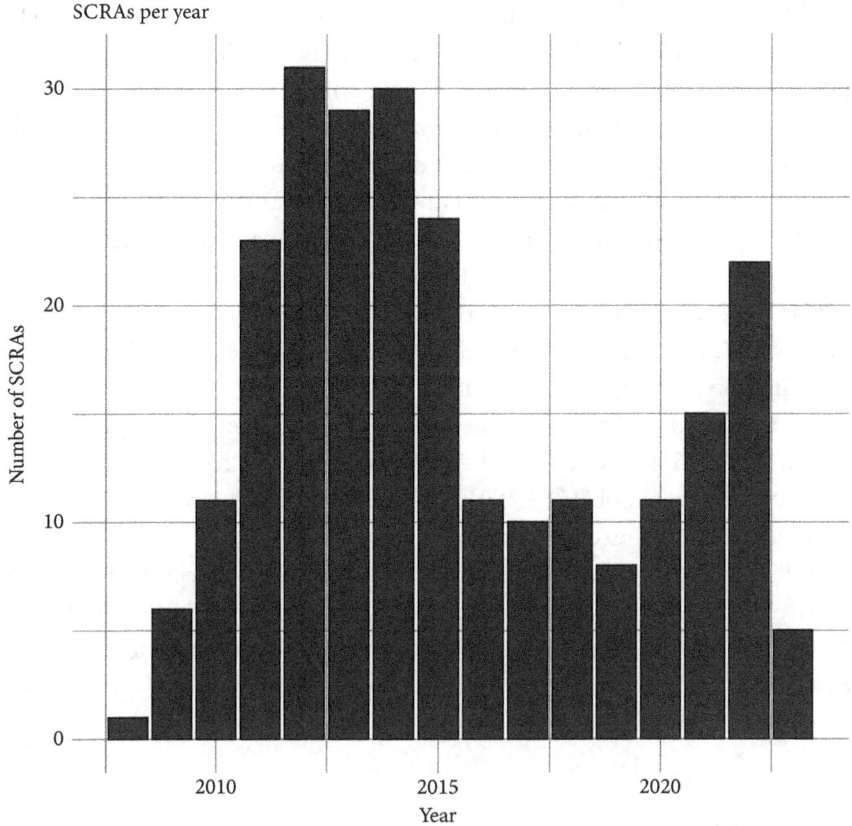

Figure 5.2. Novel SCRAs reported to the EUDA from 2008 to 2023. Between 2011 and 2015 on average 27 new SCRAs entered the European NPS market per year. From 2016 to 2020 a decrease to 10 novel compounds per year was observed. However, in 2021 and 2022 a rise of novel alerted compounds was observed with 15 and 22, respectively. Nevertheless, in 2023 only 5 novel SCRAs were reported to the EU Early Warning System by member countries.[10]

5.1.3. Displacement of SCRAs by Semi-Synthetic Cannabinoids (SSCs)

As a consequence of the class-wide ban in China, a shift on the SCRA market was observed with the occurrence of semi-synthetic cannabinoids (SSCs) in 2022,[10] which coincided with the legalization of cannabis by some states in the United States. These compounds are structurally more closely related to phytocannabinoids, and especially Δ^9-THC, but have simple chemical modifications (see Figure 5.1). It is believed that legal cannabis products, such as cannabidiol (CBD), a phytocannabinoid with no psychoactive properties, are extracted from cannabis hemp, and these compounds are then used as "precursors" to synthesize SSCs.[10] This process is especially facilitated by the price drop of CBD-rich hemp due to overproduction (in the United States: $3.75 per % CBD per pound in 2019 versus $0.75 per % CBD per pound in 2023).[14] For example, Δ^8-THC can be synthesized from CBD via a ring closure reaction in the presence of an acid catalyst.[15] Another SSC is hexahydrocannabinol (HHC), which was first reported to the EUDA in May 2022 by Danish authorities.[10,16] It is a derivative of Δ^9-THC, formed by reduction of the cyclohexene ring.

Other identified SCCs on the drug market are hexahydrocannabinol acetate (HHC-O), hexahydrocannabiphorol (HHC-P), tetrahydrocannabidiol (H4-CBD), tetrahydrocannabiphorol (THC-P), and hexahydrocannabihexol (HHCH).[10]

In line with the occurrence of SCCs in 2022, it is not surprising that only 5 novel SCRAs were reported to the EU Early Warning System in 2023.[10] Although SCCs are derived from phytocannabinoids, they are still monitored by the UNODC as well as the EUDA in their respective early warning systems and are classified as NPS.

5.2. Intoxications: Symptoms and Management

Symptoms of SCRA intoxication are highly variable and often more severe than those seen with phytocannabinoids. The management may involve intensive care capacities in severe cases and depending from the organ system affected.

5.2.1. Intoxication and Adverse Effects

Different characteristics affect the toxicity of a compound. First, the toxicity of a substance depends on the route of administration (e.g., distribution in the body) and on pharmacokinetic properties (e.g., lipophilicity). The toxicity of SCRAs therefore depends on whether they are ingested by smoking (herbal blends, resin), inhalation (e-liquids), insufflation (powders), or orally (edibles). SCCs also can be consumed via these routes but are often ingested as edibles in the form of sweets[10] or candy that have been marketed, which can lead to accidental intoxications of children[17,18] who unknowingly consume these products. Second, the pharmacodynamic ability to bind and activate a particular receptor, known as the receptor binding affinity (Ki), plays an important role for the toxicity of a specific substance.*

Cannabinoids target the two identified cannabinoid receptors CB_1 and CB_2, which are both G-protein-coupled receptors (GPCRs).[19] CB_1 receptors are primarily located in central and peripheral neurons, especially in the hippocampus, basal ganglia, cortex, amygdala, and cerebellum,[20] whereas CB_2 receptors are mainly present in cells from the immune system.[19,21] CB_1 is known for managing the psychoactive and behavioral effects of cannabinoids. Compared to Δ^9-THC (human Ki = 36.64 nM),[22] which is a partial CB_1 agonist, SCRAs can be full CB_1 agonists with both receptor affinity as well as activity in the low nanomolar range (e.g., MDMB-4en-PICA $hK_i = 0.28$ nM; CP-55,940 $hK_i = 1.2$ nM).[23]

Hence, serious neuropsychiatric toxicity and potential adverse effects compared with cannabis are possible and have been reported in the literature.

Wolfe et al.[24] found in their study on the relationship of recreational drug consumption and seizures a significant association between SCRAs consumption and a higher seizure incidence (odds ratio [OR] 2.90; 95% confidence interval [CI] 2.19–3.84). Further, they observed a lower seizure incidence for cannabis (OR 0.65; 95% CI 0.50–0.86) and other classic drugs of abuse.

Anderson et al.[25] investigated neuropsychiatric presentation of adolescents (age 13–19) with SCRA-related intoxication presented in an emergency room compared to traditional cannabis exposure. Adolescents with confirmed mono-SCRA consumption had higher odds of coma and/or central nervous system depression (OR 3.42; 95% CI 1.51–7.75) and seizures OR 3.89; 95% CI 1.39–10.94) when compared with the cannabis-only group. Further, SCRA-polydrug users had higher odds for both agitation (OR 3.11;

* The interaction of the compound with the receptor can be agonistic or antagonistic. Agonists activate the receptor functions after binding and can be differentiated into full agonists, partial agonists, and inverse agonists. The effect of the compound can be described by its potency and efficacy. Potency is the amount of compound needed to produce a specific effect, often described by the concentration of the compound that produces 50% of its maximum effect (EC_{50}). The efficacy (E_{max}) refers to the extent to which a compound can activate a specific receptor signaling pathway. Antagonists are defined as substrates, which bind to the receptor without activating its functions and, at the same time, block the binding of an agonist to the receptor.

95% CI 1.56–7.44) and seizures (OR 4.8; 95% CI 1.80–12.74) compared with cannabis-polydrug exposures.

In a prospective observational study (data from 2013–2020) by the Poison-Information Centre Freiburg (Germany) of patients (*n* = 48) treated in emergency departments after NPS consumption, 12 different SCRAs were identified and quantified in a concentration range of 0.04 ng/mL (MDMB-CHMICA) to 45 ng/mL (5F-MDMB-PICA).[26] Of these 48 cases, 44 had confirmed polydrug use, which could be multiple SCRAs or other classic drugs of abuse. A wide variety of clinical symptoms were reported for these non-fatal SCRA intoxications, including tachycardia (*n* = 16), nausea/vomiting (*n* = 14), epileptic seizure (*n* = 12), agitation (*n* = 10), disorientation (*n* = 10), hallucinations (*n* = 9), mydriasis (*n* = 7), respiratory symptoms (*n* = 7), bradycardia (*n* = 6), trembling (*n* = 6), pain (*n* = 6), hypotension (*n* = 5), withdrawal (*n* = 5), hypertension (*n* = 5), syncope (*n* = 4), anxiety (*n* = 3), dizziness (*n* = 3), paleness (*n* = 3), and ataxia (*n* = 3). Janssens et al.[26] also observed for more potent SCRAs lower SCRA concentrations in serum samples, which confirms that lower doses of SCRAs are required to produce psychoactive effects; this presents further challenges for their forensic toxicological detection.

Since SCCs are structurally closely related to Δ^9-THC, a partial CB_1 agonist, it is not surprising that these novel compounds also have lower receptor affinities and activities compared to third- and fourth-generation SCRAs. Furthermore, it is worth noting that SCC's (*S*) and (*R*)-epimers have been shown to exhibit different CB_1 activities.[18,26]

Labadie et al.[27] conducted a retrospective observational study of self-reported cases of HHC (hexahydrocannabinol) intoxications from calls to French poison centers between January 1, 2022, to May 31, 2023. Of the 37 included cases, the following Poisoning Severity Scores (PSS) were observed: minor (PSS 1) in 15 patients (40%); moderate (PSS 2) in 15 patients (43%); and severe (PSS 3) in 2 patients (5%). No fatal intoxications (PSS 4) were recorded in this study. However, only for 26 patients (70%) was the outcome/recovery known. The mean time from consumption to symptom onset (known for *n* = 18) was 101 minutes (range 10–240 min). Symptoms varied among the 37 patients, including neurological (*n* = 28), cardiovascular (*n* = 20), gastrointestinal (*n* = 11), psychiatric (*n* = 9), ophthalmological (*n* = 7), respiratory (*n* = 5), mucocutaneous (*n* = 4), urinary (*n* = 1), and other (*n* = 9, asthenia, muscle pain, excessive sweating) symptoms. Twenty-four patients (64%) required medical treatment and 13 patients (35%) were monitored at home by their families. Of the 24 patients who received medical treatment, 22 were admitted to a hospital and received medical assessment, clinical monitoring, and symptomatic treatment. Only one patient needed the administration of sedatives because of intense agitation.

To the best of the authors' knowledge, up to this date no fatal intoxications have been reported after SCC consumption.

5.2.2. Management of Intoxication

The management of an acute intoxication typically involves supportive care, which includes administering intravenous fluids and electrolyte supplementation if needed. Treatment of specific organ failure due to SCRA use (e.g., renal failure, cardiac arrest) should be treated with reference to the actual existing international guidelines of each specialization. Benzodiazepines are commonly used to treat symptoms such as irritability, agitation, anxiety, and seizures, while antiemetics are occasionally used for hyperemesis. For severe symptoms such as acute psychosis, agitation, or mania with psychotic features, antipsychotics (e.g., haloperidol) should be prescribed. Quetiapine also has been found useful in treating acute withdrawal symptoms when benzodiazepine treatment alone has been insufficient.

5.3. Chronic Use, Long-Term Adverse Health Effects

In general, the knowledge on adverse long-term health outcomes of SCRA is limited, as well as the general awareness regarding the damaging potential of these drugs. Although comparable to the desirable psychotropic effects of herbal cannabis, the adverse health effects of SCRA seem to be more intense in terms of duration and severity. In contrast to herbal cannabis, SCRAs have been found to produce additional and specific undesired effects, ranging in intensity from mild vegetative distress to severe psychomotor agitation or various organ dysfunctions (see section 5.3.1). Often, it is unknown whether acute SCRA adverse health effects result from a single or rare use or from regular and chronic abuse.

5.3.1. Physical Adverse Events (AEs) Due to SCRA Consumption

Physical AEs related to SCRA abuse are well described and mainly concern the cardiovascular and renal system as well as the liver. However, the current literature mainly consists of case reports, involving especially acute effects from intoxications, which are often hard to distinguish from the consequences of chronic long-term abuse of SCRAs. In general, abuse or intoxication with SCRAs can trigger severe multisystemic organ damage, which potentially is fatal. The different causal mechanisms have not been described exactly and may vary in the different organ systems. Overall, toxicity associated with SCRAs probably is mediated by activating cannabinoids (CB_1 and CB_2 receptor) and non-cannabinoids targets (e.g., G-protein-coupled receptor R55 [GPR55]), increasing the levels of reactive oxygenic species (ROS) and inflammatory cytokines and disturbing anti-inflammatory and antioxidant mechanisms. Here we describe acute and long-term effects in the most relevant organ systems and their probable pathophysiology.

5.3.1.1. Cardiovascular Complications

SCRAs can lead to multiple cardiovascular issues, with hypertension and tachycardia being the most commonly reported side effects (see section 5.2.1). However, more severe cardiac adverse events, including various arrhythmias such as sinus bradycardia, atrioventricular blockage, as well as ventricular and atrial fibrillation, have been linked to SCRA use. Cases of acute myocardial ischemia and cardiac arrest, particularly in adolescents and young adults, as well as several fatalities, have been documented following the use of SCRAs. The most probable causative mechanism is assumed to be an interaction of SCRAs with cardiac CB_1 receptor, leading to an activation of various kinase proteins (e.g., mitogen-activated protein kinase [MAPKs]), which trigger a subsequent apoptotic signaling pathway. Further, the consumption of SCRAs may severely impair mitochondrial function, resulting in fatal oxidative stress leading to myocardial damage with a high risk of mortality. Finally, cardiovascular adverse events among SCRA consumers may also result directly from CB_1 receptor activation in the heart, with the consequence of severe activation of the sympathetic nervous system and inhibition of the parasympathetic nervous system.

5.3.1.2. Renal Complications

Although renal toxicity is uncommon with SCRA use, growing evidence suggests that cannabis and its synthetic analogues may adversely affect kidney function, even in healthy individuals. Numerous case reports have linked SCRA ingestion to acute kidney injury in healthy adolescents and adults with no prior history of renal disease. These individuals typically present to the emergency department with symptoms such as severe nausea, vomiting, and gastrointestinal or flank pain, along with elevated creatinine and urea levels. Some cases have shown acute tubular necrosis and interstitial nephritis upon kidney biopsy. Although the exact pathophysiology of kidney damage is unknown, it is obvious that SCRAs may disturb endocannabinoid-mediated renal homeostasis by stimulation of the CB_1 and CB_2 receptors. In vitro studies have also demonstrated mitochondrial damage and induction of oxidative stress by various SCRAs.

5.3.1.3. Liver Complications

Patients with a history of chronic SCRA use often experience toxic hepatitis and present symptoms such as abdominal pain, vomiting, and fatigue. In the laboratory, elevated liver enzymes can often be found, indicating serious liver damage. Liver failure is a common cause of death among SCRA users. The exact mechanism of SCRA-induced hepatotoxicity is not fully understood, but oxidative stress and damage of the mitochondria/the endoplasmic reticulum are major contributors. Additionally, an intense inflammatory response plays a significant role in SCRA-induced liver injury. Other suggested mechanisms include direct activation of liver CB_1 and CB_2 receptors, which are implicated in liver disease progression. Inhibition of the CB_1 receptor has been found to reduce the inflammatory response linked to toxin-induced liver damage. Overall, SCRA-induced liver injury involves oxidative stress, inflammation, and receptor-mediated pathways.[28]

5.3.2. Mental Health Adverse Events Due to Cannabinoids

As previously mentioned, the main psychoactive effects of cannabinoid-based drugs are mediated through direct stimulation of the CB_1 receptor (see section 5.2). Since CB receptors interact with additional neurotransmitter systems, cannabinoids exert their effects on a variety of cognitive functions, emotional processing, and regulation of sensory perception. Therefore, longitudinal studies on long-term adverse effects in adolescents and young adults, which used herbal cannabinoids, yielded various cognitive deficits in memory, executive functions, attention, and processing speed of information.[29] In accordance with this, neuroimaging studies showed evidence of functional and structural impairment in frontal and cerebellar brain regions.[30] In the field of psychiatry, chronic abuse of cannabis is linked to negative outcomes in psychosis, mood disorders, and anxiety. In general, higher Δ^9-THC concentration (also referred to as high-potent cannabis) is associated with more severe mental health effects compared to lower concentrated Δ^9-THC. Further, chronic cannabinoid use can lead to cannabis use disorders, with withdrawal symptoms depending on dosage and frequency.

5.3.2.1. Cognitive Alterations Resulting from SCRAs

Only a few studies have experimentally assessed the impact of SCRAs in humans on cognitive functions; compared to recreational users of herbal cannabis, impaired executive functions were found in chronic SCRA users, which have been tested with various experimental cognitive tasks (e.g., Go/NoGo test, trail-making test).[31,32] Further, studies in SCRA users found that long-term consumption was associated not only with executive dysfunction, but also with impaired emotional processing, which has been assessed by emotional face-recognition tasks.[33] A limited number of neuroimaging studies investigated and corroborated the above-mentioned findings and found that, compared to healthy controls, chronic SCRA users have overall and specific reduced gray matter volume, mainly in the frontal, thalamic, and cerebellar regions which are linked to working memory depletion.[34,35]

5.3.2.2. Effects of SCRAs on Psychiatric Conditions

The negative health effects of SCRA on psychiatric conditions are difficult to estimate since most of the evidence stems from case reports. SCRAs produce effects similar to Δ^9-THC by stimulating CB_1 receptors in the brain, but have up to 200 times higher potencies and can also impact the sympathetic nervous system and 5-HT_{2A} receptors, leading to hallucinations or altered mental states. Further, polydrug consumption of SCRAs together with other psychotropic substances makes it sometimes difficult to distinguish and assign specific effects to a certain drug.

Despite the chemical heterogeneity of the consumed SCRA, most individuals exhibit similar symptoms, including high irritability and aggressive behavior involving psychotic symptoms. Common psychotic symptoms include paranoid psychosis, hallucinations, and agitation.[36] Several case reports have described that acute suicidal crises may especially and frequently be linked to SCRAs.[37] Although most of the described symptoms involving SCRAs were short and lasted only several hours, medium-term effects lasting from 1 week to 8 months, with symptoms such as visual hallucinations and memory and speech impairments, have also been observed.

5.4. Treatment Options

Similar to other substance use disorders, the 11th revision of the International Classification of Diseases includes a chapter on synthetic cannabis use disorder (sCUD) (ICD-11: 6C47). Individuals with SCRA use disorders often report an initial pleasurable effect that quickly shifts to feelings of restlessness, agitation, and an intense craving to continue use. Due to the higher potency of SCRAs, the available data suggest that compared to herbal cannabis, the use of SCRAs may lead to a more rapid and severe development of harmful use patterns or dependence.

5.4.1. Assessment

Only a minority of SCRA users deliberately report on SCRA use or present themselves for treatment. Further, SCRAs are usually not detected in routine urine drug screenings (immunoassays), available in clinical laboratory medicine; therefore a thorough clinical assessment of cannabis and other drug use is required. Clinicians should also be aware of cardiovascular, renal, or mental problems as primary manifestation of SCRA misuse. Therefore, a laboratory assessment of electrolytes and renal and hepatic parameters should be included in the medical screening of SCRA users.

5.4.2. Withdrawal

According to DSM 5 and ICD-11, cannabis withdrawal syndrome is recognized as a specific diagnosis characterized by a heterogenic complex of symptoms (e.g., anxiety, sleep disturbance, aggressive behavior), due to the termination of cannabis use after long-term application. SCRA withdrawal symptoms may vary in intensity, ranging from mild to severe, and may include serious adverse effects like seizures, psychotic symptoms, or suicidal ideations. The severity of withdrawal often correlates with the amount and frequency used, though factors such as potency, polydrug consumption, and co-occurring psychiatric conditions can increase the risk of severe withdrawal syndrome. In the absence of a specific assessment tool for SCRA withdrawal, the commonly applied Cannabis Withdrawal Assessment Scale may be appropriate. A study from New Zealand found that the harm associated with SCRA use directly impacted admissions to addiction treatment services. Further, patients experiencing SCRA withdrawal symptoms often required intensive interventions, including medication and inpatient detoxification.[38] In the absence of evidence-based pharmacological treatments, gradual dose reduction and short-term use of medications, such as benzodiazepines for symptom relief, are recommended.

5.4.3. Cannabis Use Disorder Treatment

Long-term SCRA users seeking treatment should ideally be referred to specialized addiction-treatment programs, particularly those focused on treating cannabis use disorders. Given the limited research on treating chronic SCRA use, treatment approaches are usually adapted from established methods for cannabis use disorder, such as motivational interviewing and cognitive behavioral therapy. While these cannabis-based strategies are beneficial, the stronger effects of SCRAs on cannabinoid receptors tend to create a more pronounced dependence, suggesting that more intensive treatment may be necessary.[39]

References

1. European Monitoring Centre for Drugs and Drug Addiction (EMCDDA). European Drug Report 2024: Trends and Developments. Publications Office of the European Union; 2024. https://www.emcdda.europa.eu/publications/european-drug-report/2024_en
2. Advisory Council on the Misuse of Drugs (ACMD). Synthetic cannabinoid receptor agonists (SCRA): An updated harms assessment and a review of classification and scheduling under the Misuse of Drugs Act 1971 and its Regulations. In: Drugs ACotMo, ed. 2020:1–65.

3. Huffman JW. The search for selective ligands for the CB2 receptor. *Curr Pharm Des.* 2000;6(13):1323–1337.
4. Wiley JL, Marusich JA, Huffman JW, Balster RL, Thomas BF. Hijacking of basic research: The case of synthetic cannabinoids. *Methods Rep RTI Press.* 2011;1–14.
5. Thakur GA, Tichkule R, Bajaj S, Makriyannis A. Latest advances in cannabinoid receptor agonists. *Expert Opin Ther Pat.* 2009;19(12):1647–1673.
6. Auwarter V, Dresen S, Weinmann W, Muller M, Putz M, Ferreiros N. "Spice" and other herbal blends: Harmless incense or cannabinoid designer drugs? *J Mass Spectrom.* 2009;44(5):832–837.
7. Choi H, Heo S, Choe S, et al. Simultaneous analysis of synthetic cannabinoids in the materials seized during drug trafficking using GC-MS. *Anal Bioanal Chem.* 2013;405(12):3937–3944.
8. Norman C, Halter S, Haschimi B, et al. A transnational perspective on the evolution of the synthetic cannabinoid receptor agonists market: Comparing prison and general populations. *Drug Test Anal.* 2021;13(4):841–852.
9. Timmerman A, Deventer MH, Andrews R, et al. Waxy- or putty-like materials as a novel drug preparation for synthetic cannabinoid receptor agonists: Detection in prisons and in vitro cannabinoid receptor activity. *Drug Test Anal.* 2024;17(7):1118–1130.
10. European Union Drug Agency (EUDA). EU drug market: New psychoactive substances—Distribution and supply in Europe: Synthetic cannabinoids. In: Agency EUD, ed. European Union Drug Agency; 2024:1–13.
11. Grafinger KE, Bernhard W, Weinmann W. Scheduling of new psychoactive substance the Swiss way: A review and critical analysis. *Sci Justice.* 2019;59(4):459–466.
12. Norman C, Walker G, McKirdy B, et al. Detection and quantitation of synthetic cannabinoid receptor agonists in infused papers from prisons in a constantly evolving illicit market. *Drug Test Anal.* 2020;12(4):538–554.
13. Liu CM, Hua ZD, Jia W, Li T. Identification of AD-18, 5F-MDA-19, and pentyl MDA-19 in seized materials after the class-wide ban of synthetic cannabinoids in China. *Drug Test Anal.* 2022;14(2):307–316.
14. United Nationas office on Drugs and Crime (UNODC). SMART Forensics Update—Beyond plants: Semi-synthetics diversify the cannabis market. In: Services ULaS, ed. UNODC; 2024:1–8.
15. Ujvary I. Hexahydrocannabinol and closely related semi-synthetic cannabinoids: A comprehensive review. *Drug Test Anal.* 2024;16(2):127–161.
16. European Monitoring Centre for Drugs and Drug Addiction (EMCDDA). Hexahydrocannabinol (HHC) and related substances. In: Ujváry I, Evans-Brown M, Gallegos A, Planchuelo G, de Morais J, Christie R, Sedefov R, ed. EMCDDA; 2023:1–106.
17. Ferretti ML, Gournay LR, Bingaman MG, Leen-Feldner EW. A survey study of individuals using hexahydrocannabinol cannabis products: Use patterns and perceived effects. *Cannabis Cannabinoid Res.* 2024;9(5):e1385–e1394.
18. Persson M, Kronstrand R, Evans-Brown M, Green H. In vitro activation of the CB1 receptor by the semi-synthetic cannabinoids hexahydrocannabinol (HHC), hexahydrocannabinol acetate (HHC-O) and hexahydrocannabiphorol (HHC-P). *Drug Test Anal.* 2024;17(4):487–493.
19. Pertwee RG. The diverse CB1 and CB2 receptor pharmacology of three plant cannabinoids: delta9-tetrahydrocannabinol, cannabidiol and delta9-tetrahydrocannabivarin. *Br J Pharmacol.* 2008;153(2):199–215.
20. Atwood BK, Huffman J, Straiker A, Mackie K. JWH018, a common constituent of "Spice" herbal blends, is a potent and efficacious cannabinoid CB receptor agonist. *Br J Pharmacol.* 2010;160(3):585–593.
21. Pertwee RG. Pharmacology of cannabinoid CB1 and CB2 receptors. *Pharmacol Ther.* 1997;74(2):129–180.

22. Rosenthaler S, Pohn B, Kolmanz C, et al. Differences in receptor binding affinity of several phytocannabinoids do not explain their effects on neural cell cultures. *Neurotoxicol Teratol.* 2014;46:49–56.
23. Pike E, Grafinger KE, Cannaert A, et al. Systematic evaluation of a panel of 30 synthetic cannabinoid receptor agonists structurally related to MMB-4en-PICA, MDMB-4en-PINACA, ADB-4en-PINACA, and MMB-4CN-BUTINACA using a combination of binding and different CB1 receptor activation assays: Part I—Synthesis, analytical characterization, and binding affinity for human CB1 receptors. *Drug Test Anal.* 2021;13(7):1383–1401.
24. Wolfe CE, Wood DM, Dines A, et al. Seizures as a complication of recreational drug use: Analysis of the Euro-DEN Plus data-set. *Neurotoxicology.* 2019;73:183–187.
25. Anderson SAR, Oprescu AM, Calello DP, et al. Neuropsychiatric sequelae in adolescents with acute synthetic cannabinoid toxicity. *Pediatrics.* 2019;144(2):1–7.
26. Janssens LK, Van Uytfanghe K, Williams JB, Hering KW, Iula DM, Stove CP. Investigation of the intrinsic cannabinoid activity of hemp-derived and semisynthetic cannabinoids with beta-arrestin2 recruitment assays-and how this matters for the harm potential of seized drugs. *Arch Toxicol.* 2024;98(8):2619–2630.
27. Labadie M, Nardon A, Castaing N, et al. Hexahydrocannabinol poisoning reported to French poison centres. *Clin Toxicol (Phila).* 2024;62(2):112–119.
28. Alzu'bi A, Almahasneh F, Khasawneh R, Abu-El-Rub E, Baker WB, Al-Zoubi RM. The synthetic cannabinoids menace: A review of health risks and toxicity. *Eur J Med Res.* 2024;29(1):49.
29. Scott JC. Impact of adolescent cannabis use on neurocognitive and brain development. *Child Adolesc Psychiatr Clin N Am.* 2023;32(1):21–42.
30. Lichenstein SD, Manco N, Cope LM, et al. Systematic review of structural and functional neuroimaging studies of cannabis use in adolescence and emerging adulthood: Evidence from 90 studies and 9441 participants. *Neuropsychopharmacology.* 2022;47(5):1000–1028.
31. Cohen K, Kapitany-Foveny M, Mama Y, et al. The effects of synthetic cannabinoids on executive function. *Psychopharmacology (Berl).* 2017;234(7):1121–1134.
32. Cengel HY, Bozkurt M, Evren C, Umut G, Keskinkilic C, Agachanli R. Evaluation of cognitive functions in individuals with synthetic cannabinoid use disorder and comparison to individuals with cannabis use disorder. *Psychiatry Res.* 2018;262:46–54.
33. Cohen K, Mama Y, Rosca P, Pinhasov A, Weinstein A. Chronic use of synthetic cannabinoids is associated with impairment in working memory and mental flexibility. *Front Psychiatry.* 2020;11:602.
34. Livny A, Cohen K, Tik N, Tsarfaty G, Rosca P, Weinstein A. The effects of synthetic cannabinoids (SCs) on brain structure and function. *Eur Neuropsychopharmacol.* 2018;28(9):1047–1057.
35. Nurmedov S, Metin B, Ekmen S, et al. Thalamic and cerebellar gray matter volume reduction in synthetic cannabinoids users. *Eur Addict Res.* 2015;21(6):315–320.
36. Taflaj B, La Maida N, Tittarelli R, Di Trana A, D'Acquarica I. New psychoactive substances toxicity: A systematic review of acute and chronic psychiatric effects. *Int J Mol Sci.* 2024;25(17):1–20.
37. Chiappini S, Mosca A, Miuli A, et al. New psychoactive substances and suicidality: A systematic review of the current literature. *Medicina (Kaunas).* 2021;57(6):1–15.
38. Macfarlane V, Christie G. Synthetic cannabinoid withdrawal: A new demand on detoxification services. *Drug Alcohol Rev.* 2015;34(2):147–153.
39. Grigg J, Manning V, Arunogiri S, Lubman DI. Synthetic cannabinoid use disorder: An update for general psychiatrists. *Australas Psychiatry.* 2019;27(3):279–283.

6
Hallucinogens

*Leila M. Soravia, Tobias Bracht, Niklaus Denier,
Yasmin Schmid, and Felix Müller*

6.1. Commonly Used Hallucinogenic New Psychoactive Substances (HNPS)

New psychoactive substances (NPS, "legal highs") aim to produce a similar effect to internationally controlled psychoactive substances. By November 2023, governments, laboratories, and partner organizations of 142 countries had reported a total of 1245 different substances to the United Nations Office on Drugs and Crime (UNODC). Among synthetic NPS reported, 15% are classified as hallucinogens (HNPS), which forms the third-largest substance group of NPS (Figure 6.1).

Hallucinogenic new psychoactive substances (HNPS) are synthetic compounds crafted to replicate the effects of classic hallucinogens such as lysergic acid diethylamide (LSD) or psilocybin. Similar to classic hallucinogens, HNPS can profoundly alter consciousness by dissolving the boundaries of the self, inducing depersonalization, distorting perception, altering cognition, and intensifying emotional responses from euphoria to panic, as well as various other effects. It is commonly assumed that the acute effects of hallucinogens are highly influenced by dose, but also by nonpharmacological factors such as the current mental state of the respective person as well as environmental factors. The most common usage routes of HNPS include oral, sometimes also sublingual or buccal administrations. In some cases, HNPS are administered nasally, vaporized, or smoked. Currently, several hundred novel psychoactive hallucinogens are known.[1] HNPS are generally categorized into three main classes: lysergamides, tryptamines, and phenethylamines (see Table 6.1). Phenethylamines are the most widely used class with a prevalence of 61.5%, followed by tryptamines at 43.8%, and lysergamides at 42.9%.[2] Like classic hallucinogens, their main mechanism of action probably is the activation of the serotonin 2A (5-HT_2A)

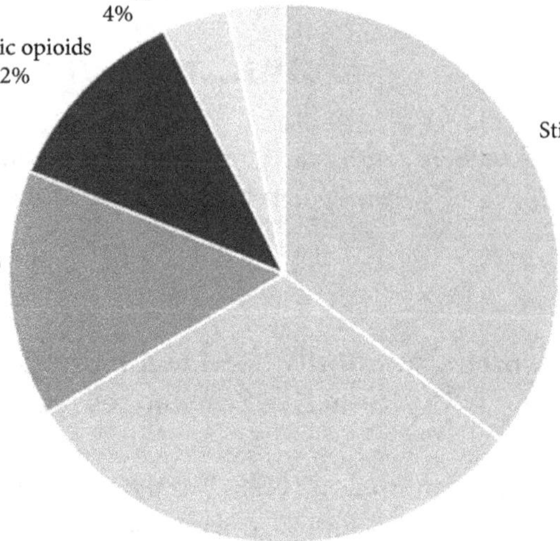

Figure 6.1. Synthetic new psychoactive substances by effect group, up to November 2023.
Source: United Nations Office on Drugs and Crime, Early Warning Advisory on NPS (2023).

receptor.[3] In addition to their 5-HT_2A agonism, some HNPS also release serotonin or inhibit serotonin transporters, or interact with the adrenergic, dopaminergic, or norepinephrinergic system.[3] Some of these interactions might result in severe adverse events not seen in classic hallucinogens (see later discussion in this chapter for more details).

Sometimes, dissociatives like ketamine, empathogens like 3,4-methylenedioxymethamphetamine (MDMA), and deliriants (e.g., plants like datura, which contains scopolamine, or the mushroom fly agaric, which contains muscimol) are also called hallucinogens. However, in this chapter, we exclusively refer to substances with a primarily agonistic action at the 5-HT_2A receptor and associated typical psychological effects.

Phenethylamines are a heterogenous class of substances that comprises not only classic stimulants such as amphetamine, empathogens such as MDMA, and psychedelics such as mescaline (found in several cacti), but also several NPS, including the 2,5-dimethoxy-phenethylamine analogues (2C drugs), the tetrahydrobenzodifuran ("FLY"), the benzodifuran analogues ("dragonFLY"), and the *N*-2-methoxybenzylphenethylamines (NBOMes); 4-bromo-2,5-dimethoxyphenethylamine (2C-B) is a relatively

Table 6.1 Classification of Classic and Synthetic Serotonergic Hallucinogens

Category	Classic Hallucinogens	Examples for HNPS
Lysergamides	LSD (lysergic acid diethylamide) LSA (lysergic acid amide)	ALD-52 (1-acetyl-LSD) 1P-LSD (1-propanoyl-LSD) 1B-LSD (1-butyryl-LSD) ETH-LAD (6-ethyl-6-nor-LSD) Pro-LAD (6-Propyl-6-nor-LSD) AL-LAD (6-allyl-6-nor-LSD) LSZ (lysergic acid 2,4-dimethylazetidide)
Tryptamines	DMT (*N,N*-dimethyltryptamine) 5-MeO-DMT (5-Methoxy-DMT) Psilocybin (4-phosphoryloxy-DMT)	AMT (alpha-methyltryptamine) 5-MeO-DALT (*N,N*-diallyl-5 methoxytryptamine) DiPT (*N,N*-diisopropyltryptamine) 5-MeO-DIPT (5-methoxy-DIPT)
Phenethylamines	Mescaline (3,4,5-trimethoxyphenethylamine)	2C-series (2,5-dimethoxyphenethylamines) NBOMe group (*N*-2- methoxybenzy lphenylethylamines) "FLY" (tetrahydrobenzodifuran) "dragonFLY" (benzodifuran)

Revised from Schifano et al.[4]

widely used and long-known HNPS and, with regard to its subjective effects, is considered an intermediate between empathogens and hallucinogens. Other phenethylamines such as the ring-substituted amphetamines of the "D-series," 2,5-dimethoxy-4-methylamphetamine (DOM) and 2,5-dimethoxy-4-iodoamphetamine (DOI), are known for their long duration of action, which might result in adverse events. The NBOMe family (e.g., 25l-NBOMe, 25B-NBOMe) is known for its potency, which makes these compounds prone to overdoses. In contrast to most hallucinogens, their use can also lead to serious somatic side effects, and several fatalities have been reported. One well-known member of the "dragonFLY" family is Bromo-dragonFLY, a highly potent substance with a long duration of action (sometimes more than 24 hours), which also has been associated with several fatalities. Overall, the use of novel phenethylamines seems to be associated with an increased risk for somatic adverse events when compared to tryptamines and lysergamides.[2]

Tryptamines are a class of hallucinogens that comprise several naturally occurring compounds. Psilocybin (found in several fungi, also referred to as "magic mushrooms") is probably the most well-known and commonly used tryptamine. *N,N*-dimethyltryptamine (DMT; found in several plants) and 5-methoxy-DMT (MeO-DMT; also found in several plants and specific toads) are potent but short-acting tryptamines. In contrast to many other hallucinogens, both substances are not orally active because they are rapidly metabolized by monoamine oxidase. Therefore, and in contrast to many other hallucinogens, these substances are usually vaporized/smoked or snorted, resulting in a rapid onset. The duration of the acute effects is short (<30 min). Alternatively, DMT is frequently administered in combination with a monoamine oxidase inhibitor (like in ayahuasca, a traditional South American beverage), which makes it orally active and longer lasting. Several novel psychoactive tryptamines are available, mostly with a medium duration of action. This comprises compounds like 4-hydroxy-N-methyl-N-ethyltryptamine (4-HO-MET), 5-methoxy-α-methyltryptamine (5-MeO-AMT), N,N-diisopropyltryptamine (DiPT), and 5-methoxy-DiPT (5-MeO-DiPT).

Lysergamides comprise the semi-synthetic, highly potent, classic hallucinogen LSD, the naturally occurring lysergic acid amide (LSA), and several analogues such as 6-allyl-6-nor-LSD (AL-LAD), 1-propanoyl-LSD (1P-LSD), and 1-Valeroyl-LSD (1V-LSD). The latter two are considered prodrugs of LSD, resulting in similar effects. Some of the lysergamides are as potent as LSD, which is already effective in the microgram range, while others are less potent. The duration of action of LSD analogues is often similar to that of LSD and therefore relatively long (around 10 hours). To date, no evidence indicates that currently available lysergamide HNPS are more toxic than LSD, which has a very low physical toxicity (Box 6.1).

Box 6.1. Background Information

- **Example Substances**:
  - o *Phenethylamines*: 2C-B (intermediate between empathogens and hallucinogens) and NBOMe family compounds, known for their potency and higher risk of overdose.
  - o *Tryptamines*: DMT, AMT, and 5-MeO-DMT, short-acting compounds often inhaled or smoked; oral activity increases with monoamine oxidase inhibitors (e.g., ayahuasca).
  - o *Lysergamides*: LSD and its analogues, such as 1-P-LSD and AL-LAD, often perceived as safer but still potent hallucinogens.
- **Clinical Note**: NBOMe compounds are sometimes misrepresented as LSD, leading to accidental overdoses. They are significantly more potent and toxic than classic hallucinogens.

6.2. Acute Intoxication: Symptoms and Management

There is very limited clinical and toxicological data on the management of intoxications caused by HNPS. Classic hallucinogens such as psilocybin, LSD, and mescaline have minimal addiction potential and low physical toxicity across a broad dose range. However, like for classic hallucinogens, the primary safety concerns involve adverse acute psychological events and potential long-term psychological effects such as persistent anxiety, substance-induced psychosis, or "flashbacks."[5] Furthermore, unknown purity and hazardous cutting agents may pose additional risks for drug users. Some consumers are not always aware of which substance they have taken, or their available information about it is not correct. For example, there are reports that compounds of the NBOMe family have been sold as LSD.

6.2.1. Mental Conditions

Common mental effects of classic hallucinogens comprise altered sensory perception, including visual pseudo-hallucinations, synesthesia (blending of senses), altered sense of time, altered cognition (e.g., more associative, less focused), derealization and depersonalization phenomena, "mystical" experiences, and intensified emotions like euphoria, anxiety, panic, or paranoia. During the psychedelic experience, most people can distinguish between reality and drug-induced effects. Similar properties can be assumed for HNPS.

In general, most treatments for psychedelic intoxication are required due to psychological conditions such as dysphoria or anxiety. These symptoms are mostly self-limited and usually can be managed with supportive care. The effects of psychedelics are strongly influenced by the external conditions and the current psychological well-being of the person. The patients should be treated in an environment that is as calm as possible, and communication with them should be sympathetic and de-escalating, and should convey a sense of security. Regarding medication, benzodiazepines like lorazepam, diazepam, or midazolam are the first-line treatment and can be used in more severe cases, including agitation. In other cases, such as psychotic symptoms, neuroleptics (e.g., olanzapine) can be used. However, these recommendations are based on general guidelines for the pharmacological treatment of agitation and psychotic symptoms; it has not been formally tested which medications work best to end states of acute psychedelic-induced psychological distress, including psychotic-like states.

There is some evidence that the strong D_2 antagonist haloperidol does not effectively suppress the effects of psychedelics and may even exacerbate negative effects such as anxiety.[6] Haloperidol may also lower the threshold for seizures and prolong QTc intervals. However, risperidone, which also acts as an antagonist at the dopamine D_2 receptor but also as $5\text{-}HT_{2A}$ antagonists, significantly attenuated various aspects of psilocybin-induced alterations of consciousness in clinical studies.[6] Therefore, drugs primarily acting as strong D_2 antagonists without $5\text{-}HT_{2A}$ antagonistic activity are not recommended. Although this is not established practice, it is also possible to reverse and shorten the acute psychedelic effects with the $5\text{-}HT_{2A}$ receptor antagonist ketanserin.[7,8]

6.2.2. Medical Conditions

Classic hallucinogens have a low physical toxicity and induce only mild sympathomimetic effects, including tachycardia, hypertension, mydriasis, and hyperthermia.[9] Like classic hallucinogens, HNPS may cause several unspecific side effects in line with sympathomimetic and serotonergic activation, such as nausea, diarrhea, vomiting, dizziness, headache, bruxism, loss of appetite, dry mouth, (inner) restlessness, impaired balance, and so on.[10,11] However, HNPS also have been associated with serious adverse events, including fatalities. There are reports on hypertensive crises, hyperthermia, serotonin syndrome, brain edema due to hyponatremia, and seizures.[3,12–14] As mentioned previously, some substances are more likely to cause serious events, including substances of the NBOMEe family and Bromo-dragonFLY.[14–16]

There are no specific antidotes for HNPS, and clinical management of acute toxicity consists mainly of basic emergency medical care (initial assessment and stabilization following ABCDE, secondary survey, advanced cardiac life support if needed), (serial or continuous) monitoring (vital signs including heart rate, blood pressure, body temperature, fluid and acid-base status, cardiac), and symptomatic treatment. Gastrointestinal decontamination (activated charcoal 1 g/kg, maximum 50 g) may be considered in patients who are awake or otherwise have a secure airway if a large oral ingestion occurred less than 1 hour prior to presentation. Laboratory investigations, including blood gas analysis, blood glucose, electrolytes, creatinine, creatine kinase, coagulation studies, and liver and cardiac enzymes, should be obtained based on clinical findings and presentation, and hypoglycemia, electrolyte or acid-base disturbances should be corrected. Fluid resuscitation should be performed in patients with signs of volume depletion. A 12-lead electrocardiogram should always be obtained, and repeated if necessary. Pregnancy tests should be performed in women of childbearing potential. Benzodiazepines, preferably given intravenously, are primarily used to address sympathomimetic activation, including agitation, hypertension, tachycardia, hyperthermia, and seizures. External cooling and, if necessary, muscle relaxation may be used to control severe hyperthermia; antipyretics are ineffective and may exacerbate end-organ damage. In clinical practice, nitrates are used for rare instances of severe hypertension refractory to aggressive treatment with sedatives and chest pain due to stimulant toxicity, while beta-blockers are usually avoided due to potential unopposed α-adrenergic stimulation, although data are inconclusive. Rhabdomyolysis is treated with aggressive fluid resuscitation, aiming for a diuresis of at least 200 ml/h.

6.2.3. Co-Use of Other Drugs and Interactions

Co-use of other drugs like cannabis, stimulants, and alcohol is common. There is very limited information on pharmacological interactions with HNPS. However, it can be assumed that similar interactions as with classical hallucinogens are to be expected. Co-use of cannabis might exacerbate the acute psychological and visual effects of HNPS, and co-use of stimulants might increase the sympathomimetic stimulation. HNPS might also interact with medication. In combination with hallucinogens, lithium may cause seizures, and it has been suspected that combinations with monoamine oxidase inhibitors may cause serotonin syndrome.

6.2.4. Diagnostic

Among others, differential diagnoses comprise intoxication with other psychoactive substances like stimulants or cannabinoids, psychiatric disorders, or medical conditions such as delirium or head trauma. Further evaluation may be warranted based on the clinical presentation and medical history (e.g., lumbar puncture, head CT scan, psychiatric evaluation). Most psychedelics (both classic and HNPS) are not detected with standard immunoassay drug screens, and false positives may occur due to concurrent drug use or contamination of NPS preparations.[12,17] More comprehensive analyses, including mass spectrometry/chromatography methods, are not available in a time frame suitable for the management of acute intoxication. In clinical practice, patients are usually managed based on their clinical presentation and pattern of toxicity/toxidrome, and diagnosis is made based on history and clinical features. Ideally, however, urine and blood samples should be collected to identify the substances used, as better characterization of the substances and their toxicity can also make a significant contribution to public health and safety.[12]

6.3. Chronic Use, Long-Term Adverse Health Effects

There is an increase in research on using hallucinogen-based compounds and their synthetic versions to explore their potential for treating depression, anxiety, and substance use disorders in conjunction with psychotherapy.[18,19] In a clinical setting, psychedelics seem to be relatively safe, which may be due to the controlled and supervised setting and dosing of known, pure compounds. However, this may not be the case if HNPS are consumed in a recreational setting. Furthermore, knowledge is limited regarding long-term health issues associated with frequent HNPS use (see Table 6.2).

6.3.1. Psychiatric and Behavioral Risks

Overall, the psychiatric and behavioral risks of HNPS resemble those of classic hallucinogens (e.g., LSD, psilocybin). According to DSM-5, these include hallucinogen persisting perception disorder (HPPD) (lasting recurring in particular visual disturbances), hallucinogen use disorder (HUD), and hallucinogen-induced disorder (e.g., psychotic disorder, depressive reactions). However, much less is known regarding adverse health events of HNPSs. Psychiatric and somatic adverse events may exceed those of classic hallucinogens. There are reports of severe and in some cases prolonged, enduring adverse effects associated with NBOMe and other HNPS, including psychotic symptoms (e.g., hallucinations, paranoia, aggressiveness, and

Table 6.2 Hallucinogenic New Psychoactive Substances (HNPS) and Their Effects

	Adverse Effects	
Desired Effects	**Psychopathological Symptoms**	**Physical Symptoms**
Dose-dependent effects, ranging from mere stimulant effects (energy, euphoria, increased locomotor activity, talkativeness, disinhibition, alertness, sexual arousal) to psychedelic (hallucinations, alteration in sensory perception, depersonalization and dissociation, etc.), and/or empathogenic effects	*Acute*: dysphoria, anxiety, hallucinations, panic, paranoid feelings	*Acute*: hypertension, vomiting, hyperthermia, convulsions, restlessness, gastrointestinal distress, muscle tension, rhabdomyolysis, hyponatremia, loss of appetite, mydriasis, tachycardia, serotonin syndrome, syncope, dizziness, hallucinations, headache, sweating, delayed orgasm, erectile dysfunction, respiratory deficits, liver and kidney failure. and death
	Chronic: cognitive impairment, depression, flashbacks, HPPD, dependence (rare), increased suicide risk	*Chronic*: cognitive impairment, neurotoxicity

Adapted from Schifano et al.[4]
Note: Not actually clinically evaluated and stated for all classes together without weighting; HPPD: hallucinogen persisting perception disorder.

agitation). Certain cases required hospitalization and enduring psychiatric treatment.[16,20]

6.3.1.1. Substance Use Disorder

Even though hallucinogens generally do not induce classic signs of substance use disorders such as physical withdrawal symptoms, some HNPS with stimulant properties may trigger compulsive use behaviors. Like other addictive substances, the addictive potential of certain HNPS may be associated with the brain's reward circuitry, particularly regarding compounds that combine hallucinogenic and stimulant effects targeting the dopaminergic system. Conversely, increased serotonergic properties of a compound are associated with a lower risk of addiction.[21] Hence, relative dopaminergic to serotonergic properties of an NPS in vitro may be used as a marker for potential psychoactive but also addictive properties.[22]

6.3.2. Somatic Risks

Beyond their acute psychoactive properties, HNPS can produce long-term effects on multiple physiological systems. The following sections outline the main somatic risks that have been identified in emerging preclinical and clinical evidence.

6.3.2.1. Neurological Effects

Long-term HNPS use may increase the risk for severe neurological complications. In animal studies, prolonged exposure to hallucinogenic phenethylamines has shown inhibitory effects on neuronal activity,[23] which may result in diverse complications. These findings suggest that chronic exposure could lead to impaired brain function, though human data are limited. Furthermore, neuropsychiatric complications, including prolonged delusions, have been described.

6.3.2.2. Cardiovascular Effects

Cardiovascular toxicity is among the most reported health issues associated with HNPS. Studies suggest that chronic use can lead to persistent cardiovascular issues such as tachycardia, hypertension, and vasoconstriction, which increase the risk of stroke and other cardiovascular complications. Additionally, chronic/prolonged administration or use of psychedelic substances with 5-HT_{2B} receptor stimulation may theoretically increase the risk of cardiac fibrosis and valvular disease (Box 6.2).[24]

Box 6.2. Remember/Important/CAVE

- HNPS (hallucinogenic new psychoactive substances) mimic classic hallucinogens but often carry greater risks due to variability in potency and receptor interactions, and unregulated composition.
- Certain substances, like NBOMe derivatives and Bromo-dragonFLY, are associated with severe physical and psychological adverse events, including fatalities.
- Adverse effects can include serotonin syndrome, hyperthermia, severe cardiovascular events, seizures, and psychiatric symptoms such as agitation, psychosis, anxiety, and substance use disorders.
- External factors, such as the user's environment and psychological state, as well as comorbidities and co-medication, significantly influence the effects and risks of HNPS.

6.4. Treatment Options

While the treatment of acute intoxication symptoms is described in Chapter 2, here we focus on the treatment options for adverse psychiatric long-term effects. Treatment options for persisting psychotic symptoms or other associated psychiatric symptoms such as anxiety and depression are oriented at the current guidelines, including evidence-based pharmacological and psychological treatment approaches for the respective psychiatric disorder. Treatment of both HPPD and HUD begins with complete abstinence from hallucinogens, alongside supportive psychotherapy such as cognitive behavioral therapy (CBT) to manage anxiety, distress, and maladaptive behaviors. Pharmacological options like benzodiazepines or lamotrigine can help alleviate visual disturbances in HPPD, while selective serotonin reuptake inhibitors (SSRIs) may address co-occurring anxiety or depression in both conditions.[25] An integrated, multidisciplinary approach ensures the simultaneous management of visual symptoms, psychological dependence, and any underlying mental health issues.

Clinical treatment options for HNPS substance use disorder apply protocols similar to those of other substance use disorders according to the guidelines, including the combination of different approaches such as behavioral therapy, medication-assisted treatments (e.g., management of withdrawal), relapse prevention, support groups, and long-term care.[26]

Since the 1990s there has been evidence for the benefit of harm-reduction programs that focus on practical strategies to minimize the negative consequences of drug use without requiring complete abstinence.[27] Harm-reduction approaches are recommended to develop sustainable strategies for addressing HNPS misuse. Challenges remain in implementing such programs at the community level, even in developed countries. Effective prevention also involves monitoring online activities and supporting innovative, web-based prevention programs to limit the spread and prevalence of NPS abuse (Box 6.3).

6.5. Summary

Research on HNPS is still in its early stages, with many unknowns surrounding their short- and long-term effects. Most studies rely on self-reported data from online communities or small-scale studies with short

Box 6.3. Practical Tips

- Treat acute intoxication with supportive care: maintain a calm and safe environment, communicate empathetically, and de-escalate anxiety.
- Use benzodiazepines (e.g., lorazepam, diazepam) as first-line treatment for severe agitation or anxiety. Avoid neuroleptics primarily acting as strong dopamine D_2 receptor antagonists like haloperidol due to the risks of exacerbating symptoms or causing seizures.
- Treatment of somatic toxicity is primarily symptomatic. Standard immunoassay drug screenings do not detect HNPS.
- In cases of prolonged psychological effects, seek specialized psychiatric treatment.
- Educate users on the risks of unregulated HNPS and encourage harm-reduction practices, including avoiding co-use with other substances.

observation periods (if any) and case reports of patients presenting with acute toxicity from the recreational use of these substances, limiting our understanding of the full range of (adverse) effects. The variability and frequent reformulation of HNPS compounds further complicate research efforts. Future research is essential to create thorough toxicological profiles, assess HNPS dependency potential, and investigate the long-term impacts of chronic use on both mental and physical health.

In conclusion, long-term use of HNPS is linked to various health risks across different organ systems. While controlled therapeutic applications may have potential, the health risks associated with unsupervised, prolonged use can be substantial. Advancing research, establishing standardized toxicology testing are crucial to better understand and manage these risks.

References

1. UNODC. *Early Warning Advisory on New Psychoactive Substances: NPS Substance Groups*. 2023. United Nations Office on Drugs and Crime. https://www.unodc.org/LSS/SubstanceGroup/GroupsDashboard?testType=NPS
2. Mallaroni P, Mason N, Vinckenbosch F, Ramaekers J. The use patterns of novel psychedelics: Experiential fingerprints of substituted phenethylamines, tryptamines and lysergamides. *Psychopharmacology*. 2022;239(6):1783–1796.
3. Luethi D, Liechti ME. Designer drugs: Mechanism of action and adverse effects. *Arch Toxicol*. 2020;94(4):1085–1133.

4. Schifano F, Napoletano F, Chiappini S, et al. New psychoactive substances (NPS), psychedelic experiences and dissociation: Clinical and clinical pharmacological issues. *Curr Addict Rep*. 2019;6:140–152.
5. Keeler, M. Chlorpromazine antagonism of psilocybin effect. *Int J Neuropsychiatry*. 1967;3(1):66–+.
6. Vollenweider FX, Vollenweider-Scherpenhuyzen MF, Bäbler A, Vogel H, Hell D. Psilocybin induces schizophrenia-like psychosis in humans via a serotonin-2 agonist action. *Neuroreport*. 1998;9(17):3897–3902.
7. Becker AM, Klaiber A, Holze F, et al. Ketanserin reverses the acute response to LSD in a randomized, double-blind, placebo-controlled, crossover study in healthy participants. *Int J Neuropsychopharmacol*. 2023;26(2):97–106.
8. Holze F, Vizeli P, Ley L, et al. Acute dose-dependent effects of lysergic acid diethylamide in a double-blind placebo-controlled study in healthy subjects. *Neuropsychopharmacology*. 2021;46(3):537–544.
9. Nichols DE. Psychedelics. *Pharmacol Rev*. 2016;68(2):264–355. https://doi.org/10.1124/pr.115.011478
10. Schifano F, Napoletano F, Chiappini S, et al. New/emerging psychoactive substances and associated psychopathological consequences. *Psychol Med*. 2021;51(1):30–42.
11. Schifano F, Orsolini L, Papanti D, Corkery J. NPS: Medical consequences associated with their intake. In: Neuropharmacology of New Psychoactive Substances (NPS): The Science Behind the Headlines. 2017:351–380.
12. Liechti ME. Novel psychoactive substances (designer drugs): Overview and pharmacology of modulators of monoamine signalling. *Swiss Med Weekly*. 2015;145:w14043.
13. Mohr AL, Logan BK, Fogarty MF, et al. Reports of adverse events associated with use of novel psychoactive substances, 2017–2020: A review. *J Anal Toxicol*. 2022;46(6):e116–e185.
14. Zawilska JB, Kacela M, Adamowicz P. NBOMes: Highly potent and toxic alternatives of LSD. *Front Neurosci*. 2020;14:78.
15. Erickson TB, Thompson TM, Lu JJ. The approach to the patient with an unknown overdose. *Emerg Med Clin N Am*. 2007;25(2):249–281.
16. Nikolaou P, Papoutsis I, Stefanidou M, Spiliopoulou C, Athanaselis S. 2C-I-NBOMe, an "N-bomb" that kills with "Smiles": Toxicological and legislative aspects. *Drug Chem Toxicol*. 2015;38(1):113–119.
17. Grafinger KE, Liechti ME, Liakoni E. Clinical value of analytical testing in patients presenting with new psychoactive substances intoxication. *Br J Clin Pharmacol*. 2020;86(3):429–436.
18. Reiff CM, Richman EE, Nemeroff CB, et al. Psychedelics and psychedelic-assisted psychotherapy. *Am J Psychiatry*, 2020;177(5):391–410.
19. Thomas K, Malcolm B, Lastra D. Psilocybin-assisted therapy: A review of a novel treatment for psychiatric disorders. *J Psychoact Drugs*. 2017;49(5):446–455.
20. Taflaj B, La Maida N, Tittarelli R, Di Trana A, D'Acquarica I. New psychoactive substances toxicity: A systematic review of acute and chronic psychiatric effects. *Int J Mol Sci*. 2024;25(17):9484.
21. Wee S, Anderson KG, Baumann MH, Rothman RB, Blough BE, Woolverton WL. Relationship between the serotonergic activity and reinforcing effects of a series of amphetamine analogs. *J Pharmacol Exp Ther*. 2005;313(2):848–854.
22. Simmler L, Buser T, Donzelli M, et al. Pharmacological characterization of designer cathinones in vitro. *Br J Pharmacol*. 2013;168(2):458–470.
23. Zwartsen A, Hondebrink L, Westerink RH. Neurotoxicity screening of new psychoactive substances (NPS): Effects on neuronal activity in rat cortical cultures using microelectrode arrays (MEA). *Neurotoxicology*. 2018;66:87–97.
24. Rouaud A, Calder AE, Hasler G. Microdosing psychedelics and the risk of cardiac fibrosis and valvulopathy: Comparison to known cardiotoxins. *J Psychopharmacol*. 2024;38(3):217–224.

25. Hermle L, Simon M, Ruchsow M, Geppert M. Hallucinogen-persisting perception disorder. *Ther Adv Psychopharmacol.* 2012;2(5):199–205.
26. Rinaldi R, Bersani G, Marinelli E, Zaami S. The rise of new psychoactive substances and psychiatric implications: A wide-ranging, multifaceted challenge that needs far-reaching common legislative strategies. *Hum Psychopharmacol Clin Exp.* 2020;35(3):e2727.
27. Awuchi CG, Aja MP, Mitaki NB, et al. New psychoactive substances: Major groups, laboratory testing challenges, public health concerns, and community-based solutions. *J Chem.* 2023;2023(1):5852315.

7

Depressant NPS—Synthetic Opioids

Vinzenz K. Schmid, Boris B. Quednow, and Sara L. Kroll

7.1. Commonly Used Depressant NPS

This section reviews the emergence of new synthetic opioids (NSO) as a dominant class of depressant NPS, tracing their rise from medically developed compounds to highly potent illegal substances driving the modern overdose crisis. It outlines the main NSO categories—fentanyl and its analogues, nitazenes, and diverse opioids with other chemical structures—emphasizing their extreme potency, evolving chemical diversity, and significant public health risks.

7.1.1. Introduction

New synthetic opioids (NSOs) have emerged as a major public health concern in recent years, largely driven by the increased availability of illegal fentanyl and its analogues.[1] Fentanyl itself was first synthesized in 1960 by chemist Paul Janssen as a powerful opioid analgesic intended for medical use and introduced to the European market in 1963.[2] The medical success of fentanyl led to extensive opioid research, resulting in the development of numerous fentanyl analogues for surgical and pain management applications. These compounds demonstrated how slight chemical modifications could yield opioids with varying potency and pharmacokinetics.[1] Since the early 2010s, law enforcement agencies in the United States have reported an increasing number of NSO seizures, primarily involving fentanyl derivates.[3] This trend coincided with a broader rise in the prevalence of NSO use. In 2015, NSO use comprised approximately 3% of all reported Novel Psychoactive Substances (NPS) use prevalences worldwide. By 2022, this figure had risen to almost 15%, reflecting their growing role in the illegal drug market.[4] In the meantime, NSOs have diffused across the globe, though their impact is still most pronounced in North America. By 2021, synthetic opioids were involved in an estimated 75% of all overdose deaths in the United States as reported by the Centers for Disease Control and Prevention, contributing to a record of over 100 000 drug overdose fatalities in a 12-month period.[1] Illegal NSOs like fentanyl have largely replaced heroin in many regions, and newer NSOs are increasingly detected in forensic casework.[5] In this chapter, we examine the major categories of NSOs—fentanyl and its analogues, nitazenes, and other NSOs—and discuss their illegal use, impact on health, and treatment options.

7.1.2. Common Types of NSOs

This section outlines the chemical structure and introduces key features of the main classes of NSOs, emphasizing their high and variable potency especially related to the μ-opioid receptor.

7.1.2.1. Fentanyl and Its Analogues

Fentanyl derivates (see Figure 7.1) maintain the potent μ-opioid receptor (MOR) agonism of the mother compound while varying in its analgesic

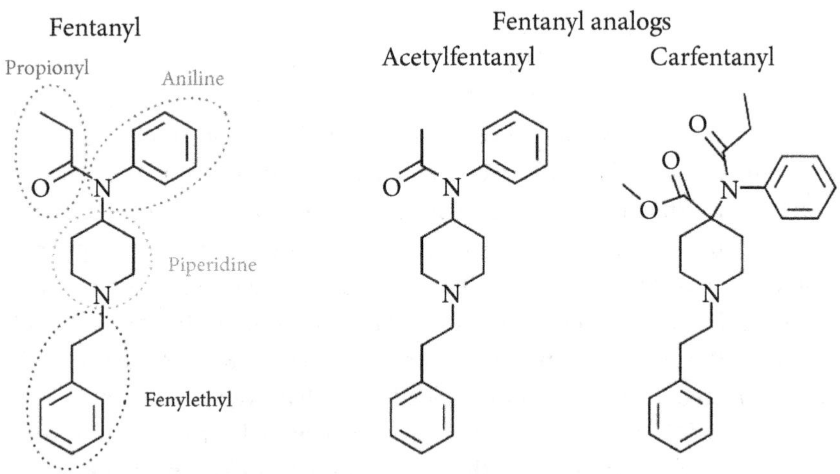

Figure 7.1. Representative chemical structure of fentanyl (left) with key functional groups circled in propionyl, aniline, piperidine, fenylethyl, and examples of common fentanyl analogues including acetylfentanyl (center) and carfentanyl (right). These analogues illustrate common modifications that retain the core phenylpiperidine scaffold.

Table 7.1 Common NSOs and Their Relative Potency

Class	Compound Name	Relative Potency (Morphine Equivalent)
Fentanyl and analogues[A]	Fentanyl	50–100
	Acetylfentanyl	15.7
	Carfentanyl	10 000
Nitazenes[B]	Etonitazene	1000–2000
	Isotonitazene	500–1000
	Metonitazene	75–150
	Protonitazene	150–300
Other NSOs[A]	U-47700	7.5
	AH-7921	1–1.7
	MT-45	~1

Table includes representative examples of three NSO groups with their approximate relative potency as morphine equivalents.

[A] Based on Shafi et al.[1]

[B] Based on Vandeputte et al.[6]

potency and duration of action. These compounds retain fentanyl's core structure, but chemical modifications at 4 key positions can significantly alter their potency. Fentanyl is 50–100 times more potent than morphine. In contrast, acetylfentanyl only shows 15- to 16-fold potency of morphine, while carfentanyl is estimated to be 10 000 times more potent (see Table 7.1[1,6] for potency of NSOs).[7] This extreme potency of carfentanyl led to its use as a large animal anesthetic, and alterations of illegal drugs containing carfentanyl caused hundreds of overdoses, often with a fatal outcome.[1] Since the early 2010s, fentanyl and its analogues have accounted for the largest share of NSOs reported to the United Nations Office on Drugs and Crimes (UNODC) early warning advisory, including 85 compounds (~59%).[4]

7.1.2.2. Nitazenes

First developed in the 1950s, nitazenes are a distinct class of non-fentanyl NSOs that have recently re-emerged in illegal markets. Chemically, nitazenes are 2-benzylbenzimidazole derivates, a distinct scaffold unrelated to morphine or fentanyl. Early examples like etonitazene were found to be highly potent at the MOR, with animal studies showing that they are 1000 times more potent than morphine. Nitazenes have never been approved for medical use because of safety concerns, and they fell into obscurity after being

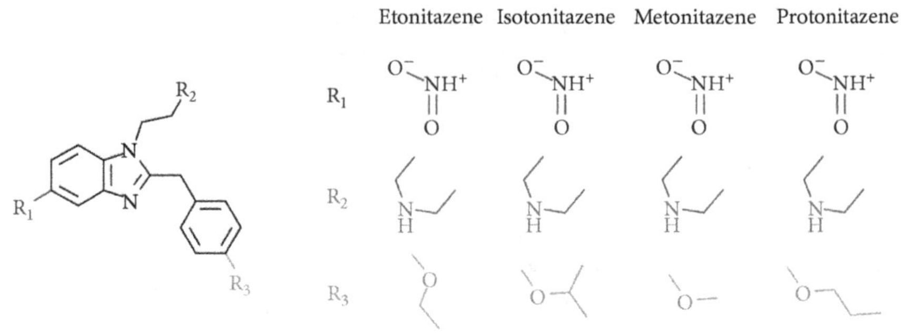

Figure 7.2. Core chemical structure of a nitazene with variable substituents (R_1, R_2, R_3) and examples of nitazene compounds.

rediscovered recently. Isotonitazene was first identified in illegal drug samples in 2019 in Europe and quickly spread to North America.[5] Several nitazene analogues have since emerged, including metonitazene and protonitazene (see Figure 7.2). These compounds are frequently detected as adulterants in fentanyl-laced substances or misrepresented as isotonitazene in street sales. Laboratory studies indicate that some nitazenes may be 10 times or more potent than fentanyl.[5] For example, isotonitazene's potency has been reported to be similar to, or higher, than fentanyl in vitro, while esonitazene is significantly stronger (see Table 7.1). Given nitazenes' high potency, even small doses can be lethal, specifically in new users, emphasizing the challenges of this drug (see sections 7.2.1 and 7.2.2). Moreover, individuals using common illegal opioids such as heroin or fentanyl often do not realize that nitazene is present. This lack of awareness, combined with limited testing for nitazenes in routine toxicology, has led to under-detection of nitazene involvement in overdoses.[5] Nevertheless, forensic reports have linked nitazene analogues to a growing number of overdose deaths since 2019.

Notably, isotonitazene was implicated in over 200 drug-related deaths across the United States and Europe in its first year of emergence,[5] and subsequent compounds have caused clusters of fatalities as well. In 2022, the UNODC's early warning advisory identified 81 distinct NSOs, with nitazenes constituting the second-largest subgroup (11 compounds). By 2023, the total number of reported NSOs had declined to 42, with fentanyl analogues and nitazenes each accounting for 17 compounds, making them the most prevalent subgroups.[4] Overall, the rise of nitazenes signals a new phase in the opioid crisis, with traffickers introducing novel high-potency compounds to circumvent legal bans on fentanyl and its analogues.

7.1.2.3. NSOs with Other Chemical Structures

A variety of other NSOs have appeared on illegal markets that do not fall into the fentanyl or nitazene categories. These include compounds from several chemical families, often initially developed by pharmaceutical companies and later repurposed by illegal labs. Notable examples are the "U-series" benzamide opioids (e.g., U-47700, U-50488), the "AH-series" (e.g., AH-7921), and others like MT-45 (see Figure 7.3). Each group has unique properties and associated risks. U-47700, also known as "pink heroin," is a dichlorobenzamide opioid first synthesized by the pharmaceutical company Upjohn in the 1970s. It is a selective MOR agonist approximately 7–8 times more potent than morphine.[1] U-47700 surfaced as a recreational drug around 2015 and was linked to multiple overdose deaths in the United States before being federally scheduled in 2016. Its appeal to users is mainly related to its strong morphine-like euphoria and rapid onset. Several analogues followed as chemists attempted to circumvent new legal controls.[8]

AH-7921, a benzamide opioid, is a synthetic opioid analgesic from the 1970s with roughly morphine-level potency (see Table 7.1). It was sold on the internet as a "research chemical" in the 2010s. AH-7921 can produce typical opioid effects but was also reported to cause severe respiratory depression and deaths in Europe, leading to its regulatory control. Chemically, it is closely related to the "U-series" compounds as U-47700 is an isomer of AH-7921.[1]

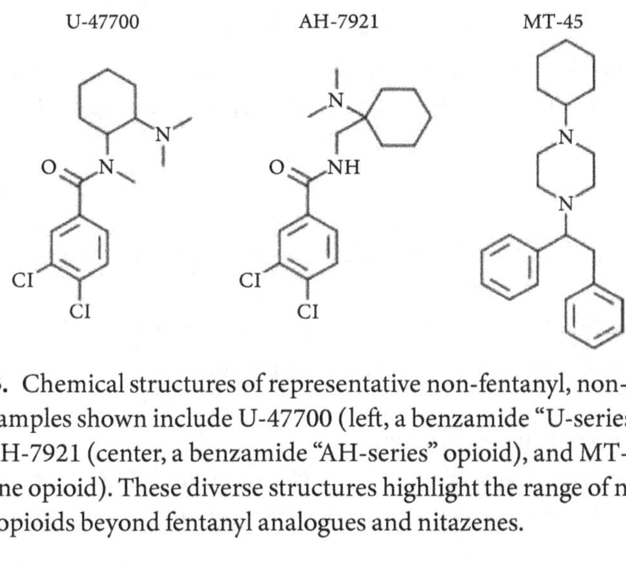

Figure 7.3. Chemical structures of representative non-fentanyl, non-nitazene NSOs. Examples shown include U-47700 (left, a benzamide "U-series" opioid), AH-7921 (center, a benzamide "AH-series" opioid), and MT-45 (right, a piperazine opioid). These diverse structures highlight the range of novel synthetic opioids beyond fentanyl analogues and nitazenes.

MT-45 is a unique diphenylheptane derivate that emerged in the 2010s. It has a structure distinct from traditional opioids, essentially a piperazine linked to two aromatic rings, and produces MOR agonism with potency similar to morphine (see Table 7.1). MT-45 gained attention in Sweden after several unusual toxicity cases in 2013–2014 (see section 7.2.1). At least 28 fatalities were attributed to MT-45 in Sweden before it was banned.[1] These atypical adverse effects highlight that some NSOs can have toxicities beyond the classical opioid intoxication effects.

Despite their disparate structures, all these NSOs pose similar core risks (discussed in section 7.2). Many were initially legal and sold on the internet as "legal highs" or "research chemicals," contributing to their early adoption. Following regulatory bans, illegal laboratories frequently develop structurally modified analogues to circumvent legal restrictions. This continuous adaptation between drug manufacturers and law enforcement underscores the challenges of controlling NSOs in the evolving NPS landscape.[7]

7.2. Intoxication: Symptoms and Management

This section outlines the acute intoxication effects of potent NSOs—especially fentanyl, its analogues, and nitazenes—highlighting severe respiratory depression, cardiovascular instability, and unique toxicities, with risks amplified by adulterants like xylazine—an apha-2 adrenergic receptor agonist and veterinary sedative appearing as an adulterant of street fentanyl in the early 2000s. It also reviews current management strategies with naloxone as the first-line antidote despite reduced efficacy against high-potency NSOs, and discusses nalmefene as a promising but not yet standard alternative.

7.2.1. Acute Effects and Intoxication

In the following, the most common acute effects as well as symptoms during intoxication of the main NSOs are summarized.

7.2.1.1. Fentanyl and Its Analogues

NSOs show high analgesic effects by activating the MOR in the central and peripheral nervous system, thus modulating pain transmission effectively.

Especially fentanyl is widely recognized as a potent analgesic, and its therapeutic application involves primarily the management of severe pain, particularly in patients with cancer or those undergoing major surgical procedures. Most importantly, by activating MOR in the mesocorticolimbic reward system, including the vental tegmental area (VTA) and the nucleus accumbens (NAc), synthetic opioids can cause euphoria and a sense of well-being, contributing to the reinforcing effects that are the driving force in the development of opioid use disorder (OUD).[9] Because of its high potency as a full MOR agonist and its lipophilic nature that allows readily crossing of the blood brain barrier (BBB), fentanyl and its analogues are fast-acting opioids with a rapid onset of action, responsible for their high addictive potential and increased risk of opioid overdose.

One of the hallmark intoxication symptoms of fentanyl and its analogues is severe respiratory depression, which significantly contributes to a high mortality rate when overdosed. This symptom arises from the drug's action on MOR located in the brainstem (i.e., medulla and pons), which regulates involuntary breathing. Users may experience progressively shallow or slow breathing which can escalate to apnea, resulting in hypoxia and anoxia, causing severe non-fatal brain injuries or death. Hypoxic brain damages can cause numerous neuropathologies such as seizures, temporary motor paralysis, coma, and stroke. Additionally, acute intoxication often leads to confusion and disorientation.[10] This state is characterized by a marked reduction in responsiveness to verbal or physical stimuli, which can impair an individual's ability to protect their airway, thereby increasing the risk of aspiration and further respiratory complications.

Moreover, cardiovascular effects such as bradycardia and hypotension are also commonly reported.[11] Patients with fentanyl overdose may exhibit a notable drop in vital signs, complicating their clinical management and heightening the risk of death if appropriate interventions, such as naloxone administration, are not timely applied (see section 7.2.2).

Other negative acute effects of fentanyl and its analogues include nausea, pruritus, cough suppression, orthostatic hypotension, urinary urgency or retention, constipation, and chest wall rigidity.[12]

It is important to note that the intoxication effects can be exacerbated by the presence of adulterants such as xylazine, that, when combined with fentanyl and its analogues, amplifies central nervous system (CNS) depression and increases the risk of hypoxia due to further respiratory suppression.[13] This combination has been increasingly noted in overdoses in recent years, complicating treatment outcomes and heightening emergency response challenges (see section 7.2.2).

7.2.1.2. Nitazenes and Other NSOs

As MOR agonists, nitazenes and other NSOs show prototypical intoxication symptoms of opioids similar to fentanyl and its analogues described previously. However, additional intoxication symptoms specific to MT-45 use have been reported in some case studies, such as profound sensory disturbances, including impairment in hearing, vision, and coordination. This may manifest as ototoxicity, leading to temporary or permanent hearing loss and other sensory deficits. Additionally, dermatological manifestations have been linked to MT-45 intoxication, including acute skin reactions and hair loss, which have been reported in various case studies.[11] Individuals have experienced symptoms such as folliculitis, dermatitis, and hyperpigmentation disorders. Sudden hair loss and de-pigmentation have also been documented, underscoring the unique side-effect profile of this drug. There are instances where users have faced severe delayed reactions, particularly concerning eye health, leading to complications like cataracts and changes in vision.[14] The mechanism of action behind these side effects is unclear so far.

7.2.2. Management of Acute Intoxication

The emergence of fast-acting and extremely potent NSOs and the increased use of xylazine-laced fentanyl derivates have presented significant challenges in the management of opioid overdoses. Specifically, the high potency and rapid onset of action of NSOs, often dramatically replacing traditional opiates like morphine and heroin, leading to increased risks of severe and potentially fatal respiratory failure, are the reason that the primary care of NSO intoxication should focus on preventing hypoventilation. Over decades, the "gold standard" for opioid overdose has been naloxone. However, the recent increase in the presence of unknown adulterants in NSOs has complicated overdose interventions with naloxone.

7.2.2.1. Traditional Antagonists: Naloxone

The morphinan derivate naloxone is a nonselective opioid receptor antagonist, efficiently reversing acute opioid agonist effects. It is the "gold standard" for the treatment of opioid overdose and is approved for intravenous, intramuscular, intranasal, and subcutaneous use. However, given their high potency and affinity for the MOR, naloxone has less efficacy in reversing overdose effects of many NSOs in comparison to morphinan class opioid agonists. Clinical studies and case reports indicate that respiratory depression from fentanyl often necessitates multiple doses of naloxone because naloxone often has a shorter duration of action than fentanyl and its analogues. Therefore, repeated administration of naloxone and higher doses have been suggested to effectively reverse fentanyl-related overdose.[12]

With increased xylazine-laced fentanyl use in the United States, the effectiveness of naloxone in cases of overdose presents significant complexities due to the pharmacological profiles of both substances. While naloxone remains an effective tool in reversing opioid overdoses, its effectiveness is significantly diminished when xylazine is involved, which may exacerbate respiratory depression and hypotension.[13] Consequently, the presence of xylazine may result in an individual remaining unresponsive despite appropriate naloxone administration.

Clinical observations indicate that higher or repeated doses of naloxone are also often required to counteract the effects of nitazenes and other NSOs. This is similarly to fentanyl and its analogues, attributed to the strong receptor affinity and rapid CNS stimulation of these NSOs, which necessitate prompt and robust antagonism to reverse toxicity effectively. However, studies also reported good response to the traditional dose of 0.4 and 2 mg intravenous naloxone for the NSO U-47700 and MT-45.[12]

7.2.2.2. Alternative Antagonists: Nalmefene

Nalmefene also has a morphinan basic structure and acts as an antagonist at the MOR and δ-opioid receptor, but as a partial agonist at the κ-opioid receptor.[15] It has gathered attention in both alcohol use disorder treatment and opioid overdose management. As a derivate of naltrexone, nalmefene exhibits a distinct pharmacological profile particularly suited for intervening in cases of opioid overdose and alcohol use disorders. Nalmefene has a higher binding affinity for the MOR compared to naloxone, making it potentially more effective as an opioid antagonist, especially for high-potency NSOs. Its plasma half-life ranges from 8 to 10 hours, which is significantly longer than that of naloxone (1–2 hours), thus allowing for sustained antagonism of opioid receptors in overdose situations.[10] This longer duration of action could mitigate the risks of re-narcotization that are common when shorter-acting antagonists are used. However, longer duration of action can further cause prolonged withdrawal symptoms, which can be very burdening for patients. Moreover, nalmefene is not as widely available as naloxone and is not approved for the treatment of OUD and intoxication, which is why naloxone remains the first-line treatment in most settings. While nalmefene shows promise as an overdose treatment especially for potent NSOs, further clinical trials are necessary to fully establish optimal dosage, administration routes, and comparative effectiveness against existing standard treatments like naloxone.

7.3. Chronic Use and Long-Term Adverse Health Effects

The following section discusses potential physical as well as psychological long-term consequences of chronic synthetic opioid use, focusing on the development of OUD and its underlying neurobiological mechanisms. The section further outlines broader systemic effects, including endocrine disruption, immune suppression, and cognitive and socio-cognitive impairments.

7.3.1. Tolerance, Withdrawal, and Physical Dependence

Chronic use of synthetic opioids has been associated with a range of detrimental health effects that have a significant impact on individuals' physical, psychological, and social functioning. Synthetic opioids, particularly because of their rapid onset of action and strong MOR agonism, possess a high addictive potential. Understanding the neurobiological, psychological, and social mechanisms underpinning OUD may contribute to improved treatment outcomes.

The core of OUD is the pharmacological drug effect on the reward pathways in the brain. As mentioned in section 7.2.1, opioids primarily exert their positive effects by binding to MOR in mesocorticolimbic brain areas entailing drug liking and euphoric effects, leading to the reinforcing drug effects of NSOs. Continuous activation of these pathways can lead to significant changes in brain structure and function over time, especially in areas including the anterior cingulate cortex and NAc, regions also crucially involved in the development of substance use disorders in general.[16]

Neuroadaptation caused by chronic opioid use is further linked to the development of tolerance, causing decreased sensitivity or responsiveness to opioids, which results in more frequent opioid use at a higher dose to achieve the same desired effect. This cycle of escalating opioid use increases physical dependence and further exacerbates withdrawal symptoms, resulting in continued opioid use to avoid the strong psychological and physiological stress of opioid withdrawal, maintaining the vicious cycle of drug dependence.[9]

Withdrawal from NSOs can occur quickly after cessation, specifically with substances having short half-lives such as remifentanil, sufentanil, isotonitazene, and protonitazene. The intensity of withdrawal symptoms associated with NSOs can be more severe and faster in onset compared to other opioids due to their formulation and pharmacokinetic properties. Prototypical withdrawal symptoms manifest intensely and include anxiety, cold flashes, diarrhea, vomiting, nausea, gastrointestinal distress, insomnia, muscle aches, rhinorrhea, tremor, yawning, sweating, gooseflesh, and hyperactivity of the autonomic system (e.g., dilated pupils, elevated heart rate).[17] The time course of acute withdrawal symptoms by short-acting synthetic opioids begins within the first 3–6 hours, with its peak around 2–3 days after last opioid use. A more erratic and nonlinear time course has been reported for fentanyl, with a faster onset of acute withdrawal symptoms showing fluctuations in severity and intermittent plateaus. While most of the research has focused on acute withdrawal, protracted withdrawal symptoms commonly persist for at least 4 weeks after acute withdrawal has resolved. Prototypical symptoms of protracted withdrawal include anxiety, depression, disturbed sleep, and opioid craving, commonly causing opioid relapse during that period.[17]

7.3.1.1. Hyperalgesia

Paradoxically, long-term use of synthetic opioids can make individuals more sensitive to pain, leading to hyperalgesia. Studies have shown that chronic exposure to fentanyl may alter pain pathways and, upon withdrawal, can exacerbate pain sensitivity rather than alleviate it, creating a paradoxical effect that complicates pain management strategies in individuals with OUD a swell as patients with chronic pain.[9]

7.3.1.2. Hormonal Alterations

Furthermore, chronic synthetic opioid use can disrupt the endocrine system. Suppression of testosterone levels in men has been reported, leading to symptoms such as decreased libido and erectile dysfunction. While hypogonadism is commonly seen in males, findings for females are less robust. Moreover, chronic use of synthetic opioids has been reported to suppress the hypothalamic-pituitary-adrenal (HPA) axis, resulting in decreased cortisol and adrenocorticotropic hormone (ACTH) levels.[18] Dysfunctional stress response of the HPA axis has been further reported in individuals with chronic prescription opioid use, including synthetic opioid use such as fentanyl and oxycodone, after laboratory-induced social stress. Particularly, individuals with chronic opioid use showed increased ACTH and cortisol response to social exclusion compared to healthy opioid-naïve healthy controls.[19] Furthermore, alterations of the endocannabinoid system has been found in chronic prescription opioid users, showing elevated basal anandamide levels in individuals with chronic opioid use compared to healthy opioid-naïve controls.[20]

7.3.1.3. Immune System Suppression

Chronic use of synthetic opioids can weaken immune function, making users more susceptible to infections. Synthetic opioids interact with MOR present on various immune cells, including T cells, B cells, and natural killer cells. This interaction leads to reduced immune response, specifically diminishing the activity of these cells critical in combating viral and bacterial infections. Moreover, exposure to synthetic opioids has been shown to alter cytokine production, which can lead to a shift in the balance of pro-inflammatory and anti-inflammatory cytokines, contributing to a suboptimal immune response, making the body more susceptible to infections.[21] Furthermore, when using syringes for intravenous administration, chronic use of synthetic opioids increases the risk of viral infections such as HIV and hepatitis C and B by sharing needles.

7.3.1.4. Cognitive and Socio-Cognitive Impairments

Human evidence indicates impairments of cognitive functioning in almost all domains in individuals with chronic opioid use, including working memory, declarative memory, executive function, and attention. Moreover, deficits in emotion recognition and cognitive empathy have been reported in individuals with chronic prescription opioid use.[22] As this is true for all MOR agonists cognitively investigated yet, similar cognitive and socio-cognitive deficits are also expected with chronic use of synthetic opioids.[23] Moreover, whether reported deficits in chronic opioid users are truly related to chronic pharmacological effects of NSO or are related to other confounding factors such as adulterations, overdose-induced hypoxia, and viral infections, or are of a preexisting nature, still needs to be tested.

7.4. Treatment Options

This section introduces current and novel treatment strategies for OUD. It highlights medication-assisted treatment as the clinical gold standard, emphasizes the importance of integrating psychosocial therapies, and outlines novel approaches such as immunotherapies, neuromodulation, and cannabinoid-based treatments that may improve outcomes and reduce relapse risk.

7.4.1. Medication-Assisted Treatment

Opioid agonist treatment (OAT) is the "gold standard" for managing OUD, including for individuals with chronic use of synthetic opioids. It primarily involves the administration of medications activating the MOR, leading to reduced withdrawal symptoms, craving, and the risk of relapse by blocking opioid effects through cross-tolerance and receptor occupancy.[9] OAT has been reported to be associated with more than 50% lower risk of all-cause mortality, drug-related deaths, and suicide in individuals with OUD.[24] However, since OAT exerts its activity through the MOR, treatment goes hand in hand with a lifelong opioid dependence. The most commonly used OAT medications are methadone and buprenorphine. Methadone is a long-acting ($T_{1/2}$ of 24 to 40 h), full opioid agonist that binds to opioid receptors, reducing withdrawal symptoms and craving without producing euphoria.[9] Buprenorphine is a partial MOR agonist and κ-opioid receptor antagonist reducing craving and withdrawal effects with a ceiling effect that lowers the risk of overdose. As a partial MOR agonist, buprenorphine can induce withdrawal symptoms when opioids are simultaneously used. Comparable efficacy and long-term results for the treatment of OUD have been reported for buprenorphine and methadone. Additionally, other substitution medications are available in some countries (e.g., Austria, Switzerland, Germany, and Canada) such as slow-release oral morphine (SROM) and OAT with more rapid onset of effects such as injectable diacetylmorphine (pharmacological heroin) and hydromorphone.[9] In addition to traditional OAT, MOR antagonist therapy with naltrexone can be prescribed for the treatment of OUD. Naltrexone is an MOR and κ-opioid receptor antagonist that blocks opioid receptors, preventing the euphoric effects of opioids. It can be administered orally or via extended-release injection and requires complete detoxification before initiation, making patient adherence a challenge.[9]

7.4.2. Psychosocial Treatments

Behavioral therapies are integral to the treatment of OUD and often complement medication-assisted treatment (MAT). Evidence suggests that a combination of behavioral therapies such as cognitive-behavioral therapy, contingency management, and motivational enhancement therapy can significantly improve treatment retention and reduce substance use among individuals with OUD. Specifically, these therapies help address the psychological components of OUD, providing patients with coping strategies and motivation to maintain abstinence. Additionally, psychosocial interventions play a crucial role throughout the treatment process and can reduce relapse rates, enhancing the overall effectiveness of MAT.[25] Moreover, mindfulness-oriented recovery enhancement is an emerging treatment option for OUD that integrates mindfulness practices with cognitive and affective techniques to foster recovery and enhance psychological well-being. This intervention specifically targets the challenges faced by individuals with OUD and co-occurring chronic pain, addressing hedonic dysregulation and psychological mechanisms underlying OUD.[26]

7.4.3. Emerging Novel Therapeutics

Some promising novel approaches for OUD treatment are currently being tested, which might also be important for individuals with chronic NSO use. Monoclonal antibody therapies are an emerging approach: by binding specifically to synthetic opioids, they are aimed at hindering opioids from crossing the BBB, thereby preventing the prototypical euphoric effects of synthetic opioids and further reducing their sedative and respiratory depressive effects. Monoclonal antibodies represent a promising, long-acting treatment strategy for opioid overdose prevention and OUD treatment. Opioid vaccines are acting through a similar mechanism, aiming at inducing the body's immune response to produce antibodies specifically against synthetic opioids, effectively blocking their access to the CNS and reducing addictive behaviors.[27] Vaccination against opioids has shown promising results in animal studies, with ongoing human clinical trials evaluating safety and efficacy (NCT04458545). While challenges remain, their potential to provide extended opioid blockade, reduce relapse risk, and prevent fatal overdoses makes them a compelling area of research in addiction medicine. Another promising novel treatment option for OUD is the use of cannabidiol, especially to address craving and anxiety symptoms during acute and protracted withdrawal periods,[28] which is currently tested in a clinical trial phase II study (NCT05299944). Moreover, transcranial magnetic stimulation (TMS) has sparked interest as a noninvasive brain-stimulation technique that can modulate neuronal activity. Research indicates that repetitive TMS (rTMS) may hold therapeutic potential in reducing withdrawal and craving symptoms in OUD. Preliminary results from studies suggest that rTMS can impact reward-related circuitry implicated in substance use disorders, thus offering therapeutic benefits. In combination with other interventions, such as ketamine—a drug known for its rapid antidepressant effects—rTMS may improve treatment outcome by targeting both OUD and its common comorbid psychiatric conditions.[29]

7.5. Conclusion

NSOs, particularly fentanyl analogues and nitazenes, have become prominent within the NPS landscape, substantially contributing to opioid-related morbidity and mortality worldwide. With their high affinity to the MOR, NSOs high analgesic potency and rapid onset of action are the major challenges in their treatment of acute intoxication and overdose, emphasizing the need for more research and regulatory controls. Acute intoxication frequently results in life-threatening respiratory depression, complicated by the presence of potent unknown adulterants such as xylazine. Chronic use of synthetic opioids leads to complex physical, psychological, and social impairments, suggesting comprehensive, multimodal treatment approaches. Ongoing adaptations in illegal opioid markets necessitate continual advancement in detection, treatment, and preventive strategies to mitigate the evolving opioid crisis.

References

1. Shafi A, Berry AJ, Sumnall H, Wood DM, Tracy DK. Synthetic opioids: A review and clinical update. *Ther Adv Psychopharmacol.* 2022;12:20451253221139616. https://doi.org/10.1177/20451253221139616.
2. Stanley TH, Egan TD, Van Aken H. A tribute to Dr. Paul A. J. Janssen: Entrepreneur extraordinaire, innovative scientist, and significant contributor to anesthesiology. *Anesth Analg.* 2008;106(2):451–462. https://doi.org/10.1213/ane.0b013e3181605add.
3. Prekupec MP, Mansky PA, Baumann MH. Misuse of novel synthetic opioids: A deadly new trend. *J Addict Med.* 2017;11(4):256–265. https://doi.org/10.1097/ADM.0000000000000324.
4. UNODC. *Early Warning Advisory on NPS: Summary Dashboard.* 2024. https://www.unodc.org/LSS/Page/NPS/DataVisualisations.
5. Pergolizzi J Jr, Raffa R, LeQuang JAK, Breve F, Varrassi G. Old drugs and new challenges: A narrative review of nitazenes. *Cureus.* 2023;15(6):e40736. https://doi.org/10.7759/cureus.40736.
6. Vandeputte MM, Van Uytfanghe K, Layle NK, St. Germaine DM, Iula DM, Stove CP. Synthesis, chemical characterization, and μ-opioid receptor activity assessment of the emerging group of "nitazene" 2-benzylbenzimidazole synthetic opioids. *ACS Chem Neurosci.* 2021;12(7):1241–1251. https://doi.org/10.1021/acschemneuro.1c00064.
7. Salle S, Bodeau S, Dhersin A, et al. Novel synthetic opioids: A review of the literature. *Toxicol Anal Clin.* 2019;31(4):298–316. https://doi.org/10.1016/j.toxac.2019.10.001.
8. Albores-García D, Cruz SL. Fentanyl and other new psychoactive synthetic opioids: Challenges to prevention and treatment. *Rev Invest Clín.* 2023;75(3):93–104. https://doi.org/10.24875/RIC.23000109.
9. Strang J, Volkow ND, Degenhardt L, et al. Opioid use disorder. *Nat Rev Dis Primers.* 2020;6(1):1–28. https://doi.org/10.1038/s41572-019-0137-5.
10. Skolnick P. Treatment of overdose in the synthetic opioid era. *Pharmacol Ther.* 2022;233:108019. https://doi.org/10.1016/j.pharmthera.2021.108019.
11. Abasilim C, Holloway-Beth A, Friedman LS. Description of opioid-involved hospital deaths that do not have a subsequent autopsy. *Epidemiology.* 2022;43(1):111–118. https://doi.org/10.1097/ede.0000000000001543.
12. Armenian P, Vo KT, Barr-Walker J, Lynch KL. Fentanyl, fentanyl analogs and novel synthetic opioids: A comprehensive review. *Neuropharmacology.* 2018;134(Pt A):121–132. https://doi.org/10.1016/j.neuropharm.2017.10.016.
13. Edinoff AN, Sall S, Upshaw WC, et al. Xylazine: A drug adulterant of clinical concern. *Curr Pain Headache R.* 2024;28:417–426. https://doi.org/10.1007/s11916-024-01211-z.
14. Helander A, Bradley M, Hasselblad A, et al. Acute skin and hair symptoms followed by severe, delayed eye complications in subjects using the synthetic opioid MT-45. *Br J Dermatol.* 2016;176(4):1021–1027. https://doi.org/10.1111/bjd.15174.
15. Bart G, Schluger JH, Borg L, Ho A, Bidlack JM, Kreek MJ. Nalmefene induced elevation in serum prolactin in normal human volunteers: Partial kappa opioid agonist activity? *Neuropsychopharmacology.* 2005;30(12):2254–2262. https://doi.org/10.1038/sj.npp.1300811.
16. Koob GF, Volkow ND. Neurocircuitry of addiction. *Neuropsychopharmacology.* 2010;35(1):217–238. https://doi.org/10.1038/npp.2009.110
17. Dunn KE, Bergeria CL, Ware OD, Strain EC. The opioid withdrawal syndrome: Presentation, measurement, and management. In Dunn KE, ed. *The Oxford Handbook of Opioids and Opioid Use Disorder.* Oxford University Press; 2024:194–233.
18. de Vries F, Bruin M, Lobatto DJ, et al. Opioids and their endocrine effects: A systematic review and meta-analysis. *J Clin Endocrinol Metab.* 2020;105(3):1020–1029. https://doi.org/10.1210/clinem/dgz022.

19. Kroll SL, Williams DP, Thoma M, et al. Non-medical prescription opioid users exhibit dysfunctional physiological stress responses to social rejection. *Psychoneuroendocrinology.* 2019;100:264–275. https://doi.org/10.1016/j.psyneuen.2018.09.023.
20. Kroll SL, Meier P, Mayo LM, Gertsch J, Quednow BB. Endocannabinoids and related lipids linked to social exclusion in individuals with chronic non-medical prescription opioid use. *Neuropsychopharmacology.* 2024;49(10):1630–1639. https://doi.org/10.1038/s41386-024-01881-8.
21. Karagiannis TT, Cleary JP, Gok B, et al. Single cell transcriptomics reveals opioid usage evokes widespread suppression of antiviral gene program. *Nat Commun.* 2020;11(1):2611. https://doi.org/10.1038/s41467-020-16159-y.
22. Kroll SL, Nikolic E, Bieri F, Soyka M, Baumgartner MR, Quednow BB. Cognitive and socio-cognitive functioning of chronic non-medical prescription opioid users. *Psychopharmacology (Berl).* 2018;235(12):3451–3464. https://doi.org/10.1007/s00213-018-5060-z.
23. Quednow BB. Social cognition in addiction. In: Verdejo-Garcia A, ed. *Cognition and Addiction.* Academic Press; 2020:63–78. https://doi.org/10.1016/B978-0-12-815298-0.00005-8.
24. Santo T, Clark B, Hickman M, et al. Association of opioid agonist treatment with all-cause mortality and specific causes of death among people with opioid dependence: A systematic review and meta-analysis. *JAMA Psychiatry.* 2021;78(9):979–993. https://doi.org/10.1001/jamapsychiatry.2021.0976.
25. Dugosh K, Abraham A, Seymour B, McLoyd K, Chalk M, Festinger D. A systematic review on the use of psychosocial interventions in conjunction with medications for the treatment of opioid addiction. *J Addict Med.* 2016;10(2):93–103. https://doi.org/10.1097/adm.0000000000000193.
26. Garland EL, Hanley AW, Kline A, Cooperman NA. Mindfulness-oriented recovery enhancement reduces opioid craving among individuals with opioid use disorder and chronic pain in medication assisted treatment: Ecological momentary assessments from a stage 1 randomized controlled trial. *Drug Alcohol Depend.* 2019;203:61–65. https://doi.org/10.1016/j.drugalcdep.2019.07.007.
27. Baehr C, Pravetoni M. Vaccines to treat opioid use disorders and to reduce opioid overdoses. *Neuropsychopharmacology.* 2019;44(1):217–218. https://doi.org/10.1038/s41386-018-0197-3.
28. Hurd YL, Spriggs S, Alishayev J, et al. Cannabidiol for the reduction of cue-induced craving and anxiety in drug-abstinent individuals with heroin use disorder: A double-blind randomized placebo-controlled trial. *Am J Psychiatry.* 2019;176(11):911–922. https://doi.org/10.1176/appi.ajp.2019.18101191.
29. Steele VR. Transcranial magnetic stimulation and addiction: Toward uncovering known unknowns. *EBioMedicine.* 2020;57:102839. https://doi.org/10.1016/j.ebiom.2020.102839.

8
NPS-Related Specialties

Kristiana Siste, Rama Kamal, Alexander Baldacchino, Hussien Elkholy, Roshan Bhad, Hamed Ekhtiari, Christian G. Schütz, and Sophia Achab

8.1. Introduction

New psychoactive substances (NPS) represent a diverse array of synthetic or semi-synthetic compounds crafted to mimic the effects of established illicit drugs, including cannabis, stimulants, hallucinogens, and opioids. Classified primarily by their pharmacological effects—such as synthetic cannabinoids, synthetic cathinones, phenethylamines, and synthetic opioids—these substances frequently evade legal controls through minor chemical alterations. This continual evolution produces a vast and unpredictable array of compounds with varying potency and effects, significantly heightening health risks. Marketed under deceptive labels such as "legal highs" or "research chemicals," NPS challenge both regulatory frameworks and healthcare systems. Figure 8.1 provides a visual summary of NPS classifications, with additional details available in Chapter 1.

The rising prevalence of NPS use among vulnerable populations highlights the critical need for tailored, population-specific interventions. Distinct psychosocial, biological, and environmental factors contribute to the heightened vulnerability of these groups, rendering traditional treatment models inadequate. Specialized prevention strategies, harm-reduction approaches, and policy frameworks are necessary to mitigate NPS-related health consequences. This chapter centers on three key populations—adolescents, women, and incarcerated individuals—selected for their pronounced susceptibility to NPS-related harms and the unique therapeutic

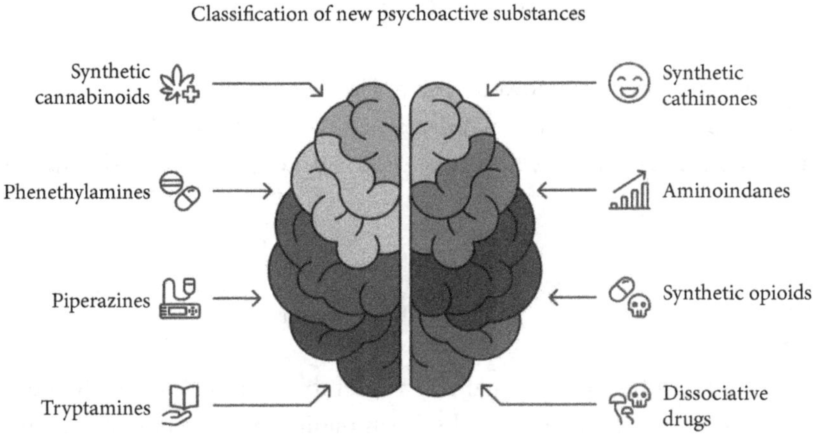

Figure 8.1. Classification of new psychoactive substances.

challenges they present. Adolescents, whose neurodevelopment is still in progress, face amplified risks of cognitive and behavioral impairments. Women face unique biological vulnerabilities, heightened mental health risks, and societal pressures requiring gender-sensitive, trauma-informed care. Incarcerated individuals, on the other hand, encounter limited access to mental health services and heightened exposure to NPS within restricted environments. These distinct vulnerabilities require carefully tailored interventions to address their specific needs effectively.

While this chapter delves deeply into adolescents, women, and prisoners, other vulnerable populations, such as the elderly, LGBTQ individuals, and migrants and refugees, also warrant attention. The elderly may encounter challenges linked to polypharmacy and age-related health vulnerabilities. LGBTQ individuals may experience compounded risks due to stigma, discrimination, and higher prevalence rates of mental health issues and substance use. Migrants and refugees, often living in uncertain conditions, may turn to NPS as a coping mechanism, exposing them to further health and social vulnerabilities. Despite the growing recognition of these groups, limitations in data hinder the development of comprehensive strategies tailored to their needs. This underscores the urgency for further research to better understand the effects of NPS and to refine interventions across diverse populations.

8.2. Special Patient Groups

Certain populations showed increased biological and psychosocial vulnerabilities to the negative impacts associated with NPS. The following sections outline these special patient groups and the distinct risks that they must face.

8.2.1. Adolescents

Adolescents represent a particularly vulnerable population for the neurotoxic effects of NPS, such as synthetic cannabinoids and cathinones, due to the ongoing neurodevelopment occurring during this stage of life. Key brain regions, including the prefrontal cortex, which are responsible for executive functions such as decision-making, impulse control, and reward processing, are still maturing during adolescence. This neurodevelopmental trajectory renders adolescents more susceptible to the detrimental effects of NPS, which may disrupt normal brain maturation and increase the risk for long-term cognitive, emotional, and behavioral impairments. Decades of research on adolescent drug use underscore these vulnerabilities, and emerging evidence indicates that similar neurodevelopmental risks apply to the use of NPS. Neuroimaging findings prove that adolescents with NPS use are far more vulnerable to neurotoxic effects of NPS because of their immature prefrontal cortex. This is due to the premature development of their emotion and reward system before the development of their cognitive control system (executive function), which causes them to indulge in risk-taking behaviors, one of which is NPS use.[1]

The availability and accessibility of NPS are greatly facilitated by online platforms and local shops, making these substances easily obtainable, particularly for adolescents. The proliferation of NPS is further exacerbated by aggressive marketing strategies, both online and offline. Studies indicate that NPS marketing is diverse and widespread, ranging from wall posters and flyers in physical locations to targeted advertising through social media groups and direct messaging platforms.[2]

A key factor driving adolescent access to NPS is the significantly lower cost compared to traditional illicit drugs. For instance, synthetic cannabinoids, commonly known as "Spice" or "K2," are sold at prices much lower than traditional substances, rendering them affordable to adolescents, who typically have limited financial resources.[3] While traditional drugs may be prohibitively expensive for this demographic, NPS are often available at prices up to 5–10 times lower, making them an attractive alternative.[2]

Adolescents with no regular income may resort to alternative means to acquire NPS. Some may exchange sexual services, while others are recruited as couriers to transport NPS purchased online to clandestine locations. In some cases, adolescents are enlisted as advertising agents, compensated not with money but with NPS itself. This recruitment strategy not only increases adolescent involvement in NPS distribution but also contributes to the widespread dissemination of promotional materials, further amplifying the reach of NPS marketing.[2]

Partly because of their availability and the fact that many are legal, adolescents commonly experiment with NPS without understanding how dangerous they can be. NPS are often labeled as "legal highs," which promotes an illusionary sense of safety.[4] They are often promoted as being more natural and safe to consumers compared to other conventional drugs. This notion is particularly attractive to adolescents who have anxious thoughts of trying something new for the first time, which leads them to be drawn to NPS. Unbeknownst to them, NPS can cause severe adverse reactions, such as seizures, nephrotoxicity, and even death.[5] The safety profiles of NPS are still not fully explored as the productions of new NPS exceed the speed of their pharmacological/toxicological research.[6] The European Drug Report 2023 stated that some of the NPS products that are sold online are in forms with higher doses, with higher possibility of these concerning adverse health effects.[7] Studies also have reported that the frequent use of NPS such as synthetic marijuana among adolescents is also due to the perception that NPS are undetectable through urine tests compared with natural marijuana.[3]

Adolescents are particularly susceptible to peer influence, which may contribute to their increased likelihood of experimenting with NPS. Research indicates that peer acceptance and social integration are critical motivators for NPS use within this age group. Adolescents often engage in NPS use as a means of gaining social approval, fitting in with desired peer groups, and avoiding social exclusion. Additionally, NPS are frequently used in social contexts to enhance sociability, celebrate special occasions, and facilitate social bonding among peers. Adolescents may perceive NPS as substances that increase self-confidence and enhance enjoyment in social settings, such as parties, further reinforcing their use within peer-driven environments.

Key Points About Adolescents and NPS Use:
1. Risk-taking behavior
2. Easy access through online platforms
3. Cheaper price compared to conventional drugs
4. Perception of NPS as safer and undetectable
5. Conformity; peer pressure

8.2.2. Women

Despite the increased rates of NPS abuse, only a limited number of studies have focused on gendered patterns of use and sex-dependent effects. Women face unique challenges when it comes to NPS use, including biological factors that influence drug metabolism, heightened risks for mental health complications like psychosis, and social pressures that contribute to substance use.[8] Women's responses to NPS are affected by hormonal fluctuations, particularly those related to the menstrual cycle, pregnancy, and menopause, which can influence the metabolism (with a lower threshold for developing psychosis due to stress or drug exposure, particularly during high-risk times like postpartum or perimenopause).[9] For instance, estrogen can affect how the body metabolizes NPS and interacts with dopamine, and can modulate NMDA receptor mediated neuropsychiatric effects, potentially increasing vulnerability to adverse outcomes like psychosis and addiction, especially with synthetic cannabinoids or dissociative NPS such as methoxetamine.[8–11] Women were found to be significantly more agitated when using synthetic cannabinoids than male users.[10,11] Women's higher body fat and lower body water content influence the metabolism and elimination of illicit substances also NPS, increasing the likelihood of NPS overdose or prolonged effects such as cardiovascular problems, anxiety, and psychosis.[8,12] Cathinone also induced significantly higher increase in motor activity in females than in males, and when administered in combination with caffeine.[13]

Women under the influence of NPS may struggle with delayed gratification due to the profound effect of NPS impairing areas in the prefrontal cortex impacting executive function and impulse regulation, often acting impulsively on immediate desires (e.g., unsafe sexual practices, excessive spending, or substance binging), without considering the longer-term consequences.[8,14] Most NPS can cross the placental barrier in pregnancy with potential for causing birth defects and developmental disorders and increasing the risk of miscarriage, premature birth, or congenital anomalies.[8] Though relatively unknown in NPS use, the neonatal abstinence syndrome (NAS) is a serious concern. NAS can lead to symptoms such as irritability, feeding difficulties, seizures, and respiratory issues.[8] Some NPS may pass through breast milk, putting infants at risk of exposure even after birth. This raises concerns about breastfeeding women who use NPS.[8]

NPS are used by women as self-medication due to a higher prevalence of post-traumatic stress disorder (PTSD), depression, and anxiety, or as an appetite suppressor in eating disorders to maintain certain physical appearances, or to cope with relational stress, stresses of caregiving, emotional distress, societal expectations, and intimate relationships.[14–17] NPS use is frequently introduced by partners or peers, potentially leading to substance use disorder (SUD) and emotional dependency; this increases women's vulnerability to coercion, contributing to unsafe sexual practices or exposure to violence, thus continuing a viscous circle.[14,17–19]

Treatment should be integrated, addressing both substance use and comorbid psychiatric disorders. An integrated treatment is trauma-informed, in addition to including gender-sensitive support, addressing the social roles, caregiving responsibilities, and reproductive healthcare that may play a role in women's NPS use.

Key Points About Women and NPS Use:

1. Hormonal fluctuations affect NPS metabolism
2. Delayed gratification and increased impulsivity
3. NPS as self-medication due to high rate of PTSD
4. NPS pass placental barrier causing NAS
5. Conformity; partner and peer pressure

8.2.3. Prisoners

Imprisonment presents an environment that, in a way, catalyzes the effects of NPS, often making the effects more extreme compared to NPS use in other populations. In prison settings, NPS use often results in symptoms such as aggression, psychosis, disorientation, suicidal ideation, anxiety, and depression, with more serious consequences. There are 4 dominant types of NPS that are commonly used in prison: synthetic cannabinoids, synthetic cathinones, new benzodiazepines, and new synthetic opioids.[20]

The prevalence of NPS use in prisons is significantly higher than that of traditional drugs, with reports suggesting it is nearly double the amount.[21] This is also aggravated because prisoners are more likely to use NPS due to their ability to evade traditional drug-detection methods. The fact that most NPS are undetectable with standard methodologies for drug testing adds to their appeal among prisoners who wish to avoid disciplinary action. This contributes to increased smuggling and trafficking in the prison, given the isolation of the environment and control in a situation where drugs can be camouflaged for screening in anything from food to a letter sent through the mail or delivered by visitors. As NPS are usually high potency, the method that is often used is through infusing the drugs into paper since only very small quantities of drugs are necessary, which often allows the infusion of the paper to go undetected as there is often no visible staining or change in texture of the paper. This adds to the prevalence of NPS in prisons compared to other populations.[22]

NPS are also strongly correlated with an increase in impulsivity and violent behavior. Both verbal and physical assaults have been reported, whether it be among fellow inmates or toward staff and prison officers.[20] Acute use of synthetic cannabinoids in particular has contributed to anxiety, heightened aggression, and assault (manifesting in self-harm or harms to others) among inmates. This may be particularly aggravated because of the confined and hostile nature of life in prison, as well as the overcrowded environment and each prisoner's preexisting mental health conditions.[20]

Compared to the general population, incarcerated individuals face significant barriers to accessing adequate mental health and substance use treatment, complicating the management of the psychological consequences associated with NPS. The restricted availability of therapeutic interventions within correctional settings exacerbates the impact of NPS use, as prisoners are often unable to access the necessary support to address the psychological distress and behavioral disruptions induced by these substances. Moreover, the high-stress environment of prisons, characterized by chronic tension and limited autonomy, intensifies the adverse effects of NPS use. This can result in a cyclical pattern of aggression, paranoia, and psychiatric destabilization, which is more pronounced and prevalent in incarcerated populations compared to those in the community.[23]

Young prisoners are especially vulnerable to exploitation and victimization within the prison environment, where they are often subjected to bullying and coercion. Some are even reported to be used as guinea pigs or so-called "Spice pigs"—test subjects for trying out the safety and effects of new NPS, as well as dose adjustments. The results set the market standards. Additionally, many prisoners initiate their first steps toward NPS addiction in prison. These are especially prevalent in those who have routinely used traditional drugs (like cannabis) outside prison and transitioned to synthetic cannabinoids due to the scarcity of illicit drugs in prison. NPS use in prison is further driven by several distinct motivations, including its use as a coping mechanism to manage the harsh prison environment, as a form of self-medication for untreated mental health conditions, and due to the perceived legal ambiguity surrounding certain NPS compounds. These factors collectively contribute to the pervasive and multifaceted nature of NPS use in correctional facilities, highlighting the urgent need for targeted intervention strategies and policy reforms to address this growing issue.[20]

8.3. Comorbidities

Other than population-specific vulnerabilities, NPS use are also associated with a wide range of comorbidities.

8.3.1. Introduction

NPS are identified to be a priority concern in public health also because of their strong association with several comorbidities, including severe physical and psychological reactions.[6] Such synthetic drugs may further add to the worsening or development of psychiatric disorders, hence constructing complicated challenges in providing mental health care. In addition to the psychological effects, the use of NPS is equally associated with serious physical health complications. The risky injecting behavior of NPS users increases the danger of infectious diseases. The immune-modulating effects of NPS are also associated with numerous autoimmune disorders. Fully understanding the interface of NPS use with these psychiatric, cardiovascular, infectious, and autoimmune comorbidities is critical for the development of comprehensive strategies for prevention and treatment.

Recent research has investigated the epigenetic effects of psychoactive drugs, including NPS, on gene expression and their potential for transgenerational inheritance.[24,25] The comorbidity between substance use disorders and psychiatric disorders has uncovered complex patterns of genetic risk in comorbid cases compared to those with a single disorder, with genome-wide correlations and vertical pleiotropy identified between substance use and psychiatric symptoms.[26] Furthermore, immune-regulating genetic polymorphisms may contribute to comorbidities between NPS use and other organic diseases.[27]

This chapter will elaborate further on some of these aspects in NPS users.

8.3.2. Psychiatric Disorders

The truly unpredictable nature of NPS, often being so much more potent at a significantly lower dose, may lead to the exacerbation of preexisting mental health conditions and, in certain cases, even the triggering of new psychiatric illnesses. Since their pharmacological profile varies so extensively from batch to batch, this enhances the inability to accurately predict their effect on a user's mental health. Prolonged administration or repeated intake can result in continuous psychiatric disorders or worsen mental health status regarding conditions such as anxiety, depression, and schizophrenia.[6] Chronic use of synthetic cannabinoid has also been associated with greater cognitive impairment compared with recreational cannabis users. This defect in executive function and emotional processing leads to higher rates of depression and anxiety measures,[28] as well as suicidal ideation, self-harm, and harms to others.[20] Other NPS, like phenethylamine, have been also associated with anxiety.[6] Additionally, synthetic cathinone use may also induce mania symptoms, which can be manifested in patients showing risky behavior, believing in their own might and special possibilities.[29] The synthetic cannabinoid users also expressed greater schizotypal traits and symptoms compared with the recreational cannabis users or non-users.[28]

The NPS classes of synthetic cannabinoids and synthetic cathinones are stereotypically linked to acute psychiatric disturbances such as agitation, paranoia, hallucinations, and psychosis. Fatalities have been reported following synthetic cannabinoid use.[6] NPS increases the risk of psychosis trigger in susceptible individuals. Several factors can increase the likelihood, such as high doses, combination with other illicit drugs, diagnosed schizophrenia, bipolar disorder, extreme depression, extreme stress, and trauma.[30,31]

NPS-induced psychosis is related to overstimulation of the dopamine pathway, causing hallucinations and delusions; and overstimulation of serotonin receptors, leading to altered perception, thought disturbances, and paranoia. In addition, NPS-induced psychosis is also related to NMDA receptors blockade, causing altered states of consciousness, detachment from reality, and cognitive distortions.[32] Synthetic cannabinoids and synthetic cathinones both increase brain monoamines levels (i.e., dopamine, norepinephrine and serotonin) by acting as monoamine release and/or monoamine reuptake inhibitors.[32–34]

The effect of synthetic cannabinoids (e.g., "Spice" or "K2") is mostly associated with presentation of acute psychosis, agitation, and hallucinations, especially if the user is known to have chronic psychosis or schizophrenia. On the other hand, synthetic cathinones (e.g., "bath salts" and mephedrone) have been associated more with paranoid and grandeur delusions, hallucinations, and severe agitation with anxiety, leading to violent behavior or prolonged psychotic status.[32,9,26,33,34] Dissociative NPS (e.g., methoxetamine, ketamine) cause dissociation from reality and at higher doses paranoia and hallucinations. Abuse of synthetic hallucinogenics such as NBOMe compounds (N-methoxybenzyl) causes dangerous delusions, loss of sense of reality, with visual and auditory hallucinations paired with aggressive behavior.[32,34] Genetic predisposition has also been addressed.

Positive and negative symptoms of schizophrenia can be seen in patients with synthetic cannabis use disorder. There are reported cases of patients who had a history of schizophrenia comorbidity alongside synthetic cannabis use disorder with initially predominant positive symptoms. However, since using synthetic cannabis, the patients displayed more pronounced negative symptoms, including monotone speech, minimal gestures, lack of interest in social activities leading to social withdrawal and isolation, lack of spontaneity, blunted affect, and avolition. Studies also found that the duration of these symptoms are longer than the usual natural cannabis use. This could be attributed to synthetic cannabis's higher binding affinity and potency at the cannabinoid receptor type 1 (CB1) compared to that of delta-9-tetrahydrocannabinol from natural cannabis. This may potentially cause a more hypoactive dopaminergic system in the prefrontal cortex. With chronic use, this may cause even more alterations in the cannabinoid receptor-mediated signaling, which may result in even severe adverse effects that warrant additional research.[35]

Although individuals may recover from NPS-induced psychosis after discontinuing use, persistent symptoms have been reported linked to chronic psychotic disorders, cognitive deficits, and emotional instability. Treatment of NPS-induced psychosis can be challenging due to the unpredictable nature of the substances involved and the variability in individual responses. The treatment typically mirrors the approach used for psychosis caused by other drugs (e.g., cannabis, stimulants) but must be adapted to address the specific clinical presentation, potential toxicity, and unique properties of the particular NPS used. The first step is immediate cessation of use, with supportive care and close observational monitoring, especially in cases of intoxication, where managing the patient's vital signs, ensuring hydration, and creating a safe, calming environment to prevent self-harm or harm to others are crucial. The choice of medication prescription will depend on the specific clinical presentation, the type of NPS used, and the patient's medical and psychiatric history. In the initial phases of treatment, lorazepam or diazepam are particularly helpful to manage extreme distress or agitation to reduce the risk of injury and manage withdrawal symptoms in cases of NPS SUD with synthetic cannabinoids. If the psychosis is accompanied by severe mood disturbances (e.g., mania or depression), mood stabilizers like valproate or lithium may be additionally considered.[32,36] For a patient who has been prescribed treatment for attention deficit hyperactivity disorder (ADHD), it is advised to stop/abort medication and evaluate the moment of restart according to the patient's status. Atypical antipsychotics are recommended as first-line pharmacological treatment due to their lower risk of extrapyramidal symptoms (e.g., olanzapine, also to reduce agitation, risperidone in acute psychosis and to manage long-term psychotic symptoms). When sedation is not preferred/advised, aripiprazole can be useful. Haloperidol is suggested in emergency settings due to its rapid effect, especially on aggression and extreme agitation; be careful with development of dystonia and tardive dyskinesia.[32] Duration of treatment in general is an individual approach depending on whether the psychosis persists after discontinuation of the NPS or if a preexisting psychiatric condition is unmasked. In addition, providing treatment for the underlying psychiatric disorders with appropriate psychiatric care (long-term antipsychotics in cases of schizophrenia or bipolar disorder, SSRI in depression), psychotherapy, and medication management is crucial. NPS use disorder can be treated through forms of cognitive behavioral therapy (CBT) and addiction counseling to prevent relapse.

Adolescents and adults with ADHD may be at increased risk of NPS use. ADHD as a neurodevelopmental disorder is characterized by symptoms of inattention, hyperactivity, and impulsivity. It is commonly treated with stimulant medications such as methylphenidate (e.g., Ritalin) and amphetamines (e.g., Adderall), which target the dopamine and norepinephrine systems in the brain. Due to impulsivity and tendency to self-medicate, NPS can be appealing due to their stimulant-like effects. NPS, like ADHD treatment, influence neurotransmitters, particularly dopamine. This can lead to dangerous practices, as combining these stimulants with NPS that act on similar pathways may lead to increased risk of cardiovascular issues, anxiety, psychosis, or even overdose. Synthetic cannabinoids, for instance, have been linked to heightened anxiety, paranoia, and even psychotic episodes, which could worsen ADHD symptoms and complicate treatment plans.[37,38] Individuals with ADHD, especially young adults and adolescents, should be informed about the risks associated with NPS use, particularly regarding the unpredictable nature of these substances and their potential for harm. ADHD patients' treatment should include screening for NPS use, especially when there is a history of substance abuse or noncompliance with prescribed medications. Except for cessation of both NPS and medications such as methylphenidate or any amphetamine-based ADHD medication, no specific regimen has been described in the literature. More research is needed on the interaction between NPS and ADHD, as well as how ADHD symptoms and medications affect susceptibility to NPS use and abuse. [38,39]

NPS intoxication has been demonstrated to be positively associated with suicidal behavior. This is most probably due to neurobiological alterations presented in dopamine transporter availability in the basal ganglia, which might be correlated to clinical presentations and psychopathological issues, including episodes of extreme agitation or psychosis, hopelessness, and anhedonia, which may lead to suicidal thoughts and actions.[40,41]

The NPS mostly associated with self-harm and suicide attempts are the synthetic cathinones in general (e.g., 4-MMC, 3-MMC, MDPV, bk-MBDB. flephedrone, alpha-pyrrolidinohexiophenone, alpha-pyrrolidinopentiophenone, and 4-chloromethcathinone) and when combined with other illicit substances. Users of synthetic cathinones report feelings of extreme panic, fear, and depression during withdrawal, along with nihilism, which may drive suicidal behavior with additional cravings that can lead to self-harm. Clinical presentation during the attempts appeared to be in severe disinhibition, impulsivity, loss of self-control and alterations

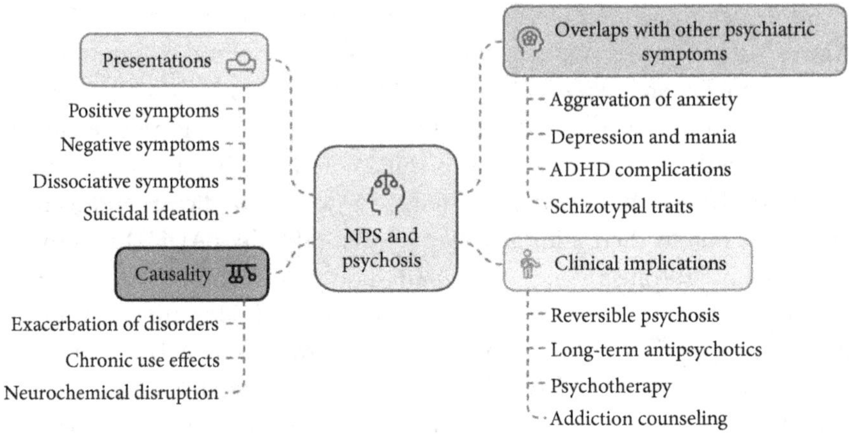

Figure 8.2. NPS and psychosis.

in judgment; therefore suicide is more likely to take place.[42–46] Suicidal risk is reported also with cannabinoids (e.g. AB-CHMINACA, AB-FUBINACA, MDMB-CHMICA and JWH-018)[40,41,43,45] and mephedrone.[44] The complex relationship between NPS and psychosis is further illustrated in Figure 8.2.

8.3.3. Cardiovascular Issues

Alongside psychiatric comorbidities, NPS users are known to have physical comorbidities with these substances, which can result in a wide range of adverse health effects. A particularly troubling area is the cardiovascular system, in which NPS use has been most commonly associated with hypertension and tachycardia.[6] Hypertension due to chronic use of NPS can result in damaged vessels, which are liable to aneurysms or hemorrhagic strokes. In addition, tachycardia, if sustained for long enough, can become cardiac arrhythmias and potentially lead to sudden death from the heart. Studies showed that ECG changes are commonly seen in patients with synthetic cannabinoid use, particularly significantly wider QRS width, lower T-wave amplitude, and ST elevation.[47] Hence, particularly in severe cases of synthetic cannabinoids and cathinones (so-called bath salts) use, there are cases with myocardial infarction caused by hypertension and sudden cardiac arrest due to fatal arrhythmias.[6]

The major cardiotoxic effects of synthetic cannabinoids and cathinones are primarily mediated through activation of the CB1 receptor on cardiomyocytes, leading to increased reactive oxygen species, ATP depletion, and cell death. Excessive adrenergic stimulation and increased oxidative stress are also concerns with the cardiotoxic effects of these substances.[48] Such effects may even be enhanced in patients who have a past medical history of some cardiac disease, for instance coronary artery disease or heart failure, in whom the extra stress on the heart cannot be tolerated. Other reported cardiovascular toxicities due to synthetic cannabinoid use include tachy/bradycardia, arrhythmias (atrioventricular block, supraventricular tachycardia), hyper/hypotension, palpitation, chest pain, cardiomyopathy, cardiomegaly, myocardial ischemia, hypertrophic and dilated heart, and atherosclerosis of the valves, coronaries, and arteries.[49]

8.3.4. Infectious Diseases

Emerging use of NPS has become a growing public health concern in view of its direct effects on the brain and because of its association with a higher risk of infectious diseases like HIV, hepatitis B, hepatitis C, and other bacterial infections. A major risk factor associated with this is the unsafe injecting practices characteristic of NPS use, including sharing of needles. The comorbidity of NPS use and infectious diseases is complex and requires a multifaceted approach toward prevention, harm reduction, and treatment.

Data from European Monitoring Centre for Drugs and Drug Addiction (EMCDDA) in 2018 stated that there is an increasing trend of injectable NPS in prison, such as synthetic opioid use. NPS are often associated with compulsive behaviors which can lead to more frequent and unsafe injections, increasing the likelihood of needle sharing and reusing unsterilized equipment. This leads to an increase in HIV and hepatitis C virus infection in NPS users in prison.[20] Studies shows that HCV prevalence rose from around 30% (2008–2012) to 41% (2013–2014) and then 48% (2015–2016). This increase may be due to the increased risk of hepatitis C virus infection in people who injected NPS.[50]

The use of NPS may also be associated with unsafe sexual behavior that contributes to HIV risk. Most of these NPS, especially the synthetic stimulant class of drugs like cathinones, heighten sexual arousals and lower inhibitions, leading to unprotected sex and multiple exchanges. This aspect was well documented by EMCDDA in 2021 in populations such as men who have sex with men, where NPS drugs like mephedrone and synthetic cathinones have been used in the so-called "chem sex" settings to enhance, sustain, disinhibit, or facilitate sexual experiences. Outbreaks of HIV have been documented in several countries as a result of synthetic cathinone injections.[51]

NPS use in these settings contributes to both sexual HIV transmission and the sharing of injection equipment. Users in high-risk settings are usually in altered states of consciousness, which will make them less likely to take any precautions, such as using condoms or sterile needles. Joint risky sexual behavior and drug-injection practices result in a dual-pathway transmission modality of HIV, thereby increasing the comorbidity between NPS use and HIV infection.

8.3.5. Autoimmune Diseases

The use of NPS has been associated with several autoimmune diseases. Autoimmune conditions arise when the immune system mistakenly attacks the body's own tissues, leading to systemic inflammation and organ dysfunction. NPS, due to their immune-modulating properties, can potentially contribute to autoimmune dysregulation by inducing chronic inflammation, altering immune responses, or exerting direct toxic effects on cellular structures. Recent studies have reported cases of autoimmune diseases occurring alongside substance use disorders, most commonly involving insulin-dependent diabetes mellitus (type 1 diabetes) and inflammatory bowel disease (IBD). This co-occurrence suggests potential shared etiopathogenic mechanisms between NPS use and these autoimmune conditions, although the exact mechanisms remain underexplored.[52]

Methamphetamine, which shares structural and functional similarities with certain synthetic stimulants within NPS, has been associated with thyroid dysfunction and inflammation, leading to autoimmune thyroid diseases. Chronic methamphetamine use has been linked to hypothyroidism, thyroid enlargement, and hyperparathyroidism. Research has shown that methamphetamine can dysregulate the hypothalamic-pituitary-thyroid (HPT) axis by increasing thyroxine (T4) and adrenocorticotropic hormone levels while reducing triiodothyronine (T3), cortisol, and thyroid-stimulating hormone (TSH) levels. This disruption of the HPT axis suggests a direct role of methamphetamine in promoting autoimmune thyroid diseases in susceptible individuals.[53]

Similarly, substances like cocaine have long been implicated in drug-induced lupus (DIL), primarily through mechanisms involving increased apoptosis and impaired clearance of apoptotic cells. These processes allow the accumulation of cellular debris, which can stimulate autoreactive responses by dendritic cells and subsequent inflammatory cytokine production. While NPS-specific cases of lupus are not well documented, synthetic cathinones (metaphedrone) have been reported to produce similar immune dysregulation and oxidative stress, raising concerns over potential links to lupus and other autoimmune conditions.[54,55]

Emerging evidence also suggests associations between synthetic cannabinoids and autoimmune diseases like psoriasis and rheumatoid arthritis. Synthetic cannabinoids, due to their strong affinity for cannabinoid receptors (CB1 and CB2), can significantly alter immune cell function and cytokine profiles, potentially aggravating or triggering autoimmune responses. Although some synthetic cannabinoids show immunosuppressive properties by downregulating cytokine and chemokine production, chronic or heavy use might paradoxically lead to immune dysregulation and inflammation, particularly when interacting with a predisposed immune system.[56,57]

Key Points About NPS Comorbidity:

Psychiatric Disorders	**Cardiovascular Issues**	**Infectious Diseases**	**Autoimmune Diseases**
- Exacerbate or induce psychiatric disorders (anxiety, depression, psychosis) - Longer and more severe adverse effects - Treatment atypical antipsychotics - Alertheid with ADHD - Risk of suicide	- ECG changes - Hypertension - Tachycardia - Myocardial infarction	- Unsafe injection, needle sharing - Chem sex - HIV - Hepatitis B and C	- Immune-modulating properties - Insulin-dependent diabetes mellitus - IBD - Autoimmune thyroid disease - Drug-induced lupus

References

1. Squeglia LM, Cservenka A. Adolescence and drug use vulnerability: Findings from neuroimaging. *Curr Opin Behav Sci.* 2017 Feb 1;13:164–170.
2. Kurcevič E, Lines R. New psychoactive substances in Eurasia: A qualitative study of people who use drugs and harm reduction services in six countries. *Harm Reduct J.* 2020 Dec;17:1–3.
3. Baweja R, Mills-Huffnagle S, Jernigan A, Chongtham N, Waschbusch D, Waxmonsky JG. Synthetic marijuana: Assessment of usage, motivation and associated risks in adolescent substance users. *Subst Use Res Treatm.* 2024 May;18:29768357241254258.
4. Werse B, Morgenstern C. How to handle legal highs? Findings from a German online survey and considerations on drug policy issues. *Drugs Alcohol Today.* 2012 Nov 30;12(4):222–231.
5. Fujiwara R, Journey M, Al-Doori F, et al. Potential neonatal toxicity of new psychoactive substances. *Pharmacol Therapeut.* 2023 Aug 1;248:108468.
6. Santos IC, Maia D, Dinis-Oliveira RJ, Barbosa DJ. New psychoactive substances: Health and legal challenges. *Psychoactives.* 2024 Jun 1;3(2):285–302.
7. European Monitoring Centre for Drugs and Drug Addiction (EMCDDA). New psychoactive substances: The current situation in Europe. *European Drug Report.* EMCDDA; 2023.
8. Fattore L, Marti M, Mostallino R, Paola Castelli M. Sex and gender differences in the effects of novel psychoactive substances. *Brain Sci.* 2020 Sep 3;10(9):606.
9. Van Hout MC, Hearne E. The impact of synthetic cannabinoid receptor agonists on mental health: A European perspective. *J Psychoactive Drugs.* 2017;49(6):278–286.
10. Thomas S, Bliss S, Malik M. Suicidal ideation and self-harm following K2 use. *J Okla State Med Assoc.* 2012;105:430–433.
11. Nia AB, Galynker II, Mann CL, Spriggs S, et al. The relevance of sex in the association of synthetic cannabinoid use with psychosis and agitation in an inpatient population. *J Clin Psychiatry.* 2019;80(4):18m12539.
12. NIDA (National Institute on Drug Abuse). Substance Use in Women. Last Updated January 2020. https://www.drugabuse.gov.
13. Alsufyani HA, Docherty JR. Gender differences in the effects of cathinone and the interaction with caffeine on temperature and locomotor activity in the rat. *Eur J Pharmacol.* 2017;809:203–208.
14. Vreeker A, van der Burg BG, van Laar M, Brunt TM. Characterizing users of new psychoactive substances using psychometric scales for risk-related behavior. *Addict Behav.* 2017;70:72–78.
15. Wright JM, Walther GR. Gender-specific health risks associated with novel psychoactive substances. *Women's Health Issues.* 2019;29(3):204–210.
16. Soussan C, Andersson M, Kjellgren A. The diverse reasons for using Novel Psychoactive Substances. A qualitative study of the users' own perspectives. *Int J Drug Policy.* 2018 Feb;52:71–78. doi:10.1016/j.drugpo.2017.11.003.
17. MacLean S, Moore D. Women, pleasure and new psychoactive substances: Gendered experiences and health implications. *Contemp Drug Probl.* 2014;41(1):35–52.
18. Global Drug Survey (GDS). *Report.* 2019. GDS2019 | www.globaldrugsurvey.com
19. King C, Jones HE. Gender differences in substance use and related health risks with emerging drugs, including new psychoactive substances (NPS). *J Subst Use.* 2018;23(4):376–382.
20. European Monitoring Centre for Drugs and Drug Addiction (EMCDDA). New psychoactive substances in prison: Results from an EMCDDA Trendspotter Study. https://www.euda.europa.eu/system/files/publications/8869/nps-in-prison.pdf. 2018 Jun.
21. Mason R, Smith M, Onwuegbusi T, Roberts A. New psychoactive substances and violence within a UK prison setting. *Subst Use Misuse.* 2022 Dec 6;57(14):2146–2150.

22. Norman C. A global review of prison drug smuggling routes and trends in the usage of drugs in prisons. *WIREs Forensic Sci.* 2023 Mar;5(2):e1473.
23. Solbakken LE, Bergvik S, Wynn R. Breaking down barriers to mental healthcare access in prison: A qualitative interview study with incarcerated males in Norway. *BMC Psychiatry.* 2024 Apr 17;24(1):292.
24. Ahmed R, Blum K, Thanos PK. Epigenetic Effects of psychoactive drugs. *Curr Pharmaceut Design.* 2023 Aug 1;29(27):2124–2139.
25. Mazdai L, Fabbri M, Tirri M, et al. Epigenetic studies for evaluation of NPS toxicity: Focus on synthetic cannabinoids and cathinones. *Biomedicines.* 2022 Jun 13;10(6):1398.
26. Martínez-Magaña JJ, Genis-Mendoza AD, Villatoro Velazquez JA, et al. Genome-wide association study of psychiatric and substance use comorbidity in Mexican individuals. *Sci Rep.* 2021 Mar 24;11(1):6771–6779.
27. Corsi-Zuelli F, Loureiro C, Shuhama R, et al. Immune regulatory gene polymorphisms, frequent cannabis use, and psychosis: Implications to Treg hypofunction. *Eur Psychiatry.* 2022 Jun 1;65(S1):S698.
28. Cohen K, Mama Y, Rosca P, Pinhasov A, Weinstein A. Chronic use of synthetic cannabinoids is associated with impairment in working memory and mental flexibility. *Front Psychiatry.* 2020 Jun 30;11:602.
29. Severtsev VV, Budanova AA. Recurrent psychotic episodes induced by synthetic cathinones in a monozygotic twin with drug addiction: A case report. *Consort Psychiatr.* 2023 Dec 22;4(4):58–65.
30. European Monitoring Centre for Drugs and Drug Addiction (EMCDDA). New psychoactive substances: An update to 2019. 2021. EMCDDA Publication No. 2021:1036.
31. United Nations Office on Drugs and Crime (UNODC). World Drug Report. https://www.unodc.org/unodc/data-and-analysis/world-drug-report-2022.html. 2022.
32. Davidson L, Davis C. New psychoactive substances and their potential to cause psychosis: A systematic review. *Drug Alcohol Rev.* 2019;38(1):66–76.
33. Perry E, English J. Synthetic cannabinoids and psychosis: A review of the evidence. *Eur Neuropsychopharmacol.* 2020;34:25–38.
34. Sznitman SR, Bowden-Jones H, Louisa K, Winstock A. Emerging drug trends: New psychoactive substances and psychosis. *Curr Opin Psychiatry.* 2018;31(4):301–307.
35. Zhornitsky S, Potvin S, Roy O, Aubin S. Psychotic effects associated with new psychoactive substances: A comprehensive review. *Addiction.* 2017;112(6):1028–1041.
36. Satodiya R, Palekar N. Synthetic cannabinoids and its association with persistent negative symptoms of schizophrenia. *Cureus.* 2020 Sep;12(9):e10329.
37. Schifano F, Orsolini L, Papanti D, Corkery J. Novel psychoactive substances of interest for psychiatry. *World Psychiatry.* 2015;14(1):15–26.
38. Faraone SV, Rostain AL, Montano CB, Mason O, Antshel KM. Attention-deficit/hyperactivity disorder (ADHD) and substance use disorders. *Harvard Rev Psychiatry.* 2020;28(5):264–276.
39. Robinson L, Rapport L. New psychoactive substances and ADHD: Implications for treatment and understanding. *J Addict Med Ther Sci.* 2017;3(1):45–52.
40. Darke S, Duflou J, Farrell M, Peacock A, Lappin J. Characteristics and circumstances of synthetic cannabinoid-related death. *Clin Toxicol (Phila).* 2020;58:368–374.
41. Oliveira PMDS, Morais ASF, Madeira NGGF. Synthetic cannabis analogues and suicidal behavior: Case report. *J Addict Med.* 2017;11:408–410.
42. Kraemer M, Boehmer A, Madea B, Maas A. Death cases involving certain new psychoactive substances: A review of the literature. *Forensic Sci Int.* 2019;298:186–267.
43. Kronstrand R, Guerrieri D, Vikingsson S, Wohlfarth A, Gréen H. Fatal poisonings associated with new psychoactive substances. *Handb Exp Pharmacol.* 2018;252:495–541.
44. Loi B, Corkery JM, Claridge H, et al. Deaths of individuals aged 16–24 years in the UK after using mephedrone. *Hum Psychopharmacol Clin Exp.* 2015;30:225–232.

45. Adamowicz P. Fatal intoxication with synthetic cannabinoid MDMB-CHMICA. *Forensic Sci Int.* 2016;261:e5–e10.
46. Chiappini S, Mosca A, Miuli A, et al. New psychoactive substances and suicidality: A systematic review. *Medicina.* 2021;57:580.
47. Yeniocak S, Kalkan A, Yamanoğlu A, Öztürk S, Söğüt Ö, Metiner M. The effects of synthetic cannabinoids on the cardiovascular system: A case-control study. *Turk J Emerg Med.* 2021 Oct 1;21(4):198–204.
48. Radaelli D, Manfredi A, Zanon M, et al. Synthetic cannabinoids and cathinones cardiotoxicity: Facts and perspectives. *Curr Neuropharmacol.* 2021 Nov 11;19(11):2038–2048.
49. de Oliveira MC, Vides MC, Lassi DL, et al. Toxicity of synthetic cannabinoids in K2/spice: A systematic review. *Brain Sci.* 2023 Jun 24;13(7):990.
50. McAuley A, Yeung A, Taylor A, Hutchinson SJ, Goldberg DJ, Munro A. Emergence of novel psychoactive substance injecting associated with rapid rise in the population prevalence of hepatitis C virus. *Int J Drug Policy.* 2019 Apr 1;66:30–37.
51. European Monitoring Centre for Drugs and Drug Addiction (EMCDDA). *New psychoactive substances: Health and social responses.* EMCDDA; 2021 Oct.
52. Stati S. Substance use disorder in patients with autoimmune diseases: Sociodemographic profile. *Eur Psychiatry.* 2023 Mar 1;66(S1):S765.
53. Jones DL, Carrico AW, Babayigit S, Rodriguez VJ, Aguila C, Kumar M. Methamphetamine-associated dysregulation of the hypothalamic–pituitary–thyroid axis. *J Behav Med.* 2018 Dec;41:792–797.
54. Rivera TL, Belmont HM, Weissmann G. Systemic lupus erythematosus in 6 male cocaine users at Bellevue hospital. *J Rheumatol.* 2009 Dec 1;36(12):2854–2855.
55. Dias da Silva D, Ferreira B, Roque Bravo R, et al. The new psychoactive substance 3-methylmethcathinone (3-MMC or metaphedrone) induces oxidative stress, apoptosis, and autophagy in primary rat hepatocytes at human-relevant concentrations. *Arch Toxicol.* 2019 Sep;93(9):2617–2634.
56. Katchan V, David P, Shoenfeld Y. Cannabinoids and autoimmune diseases: A systematic review. *Autoimmun Rev.* 2016 Jun 1;15(6):513–528.
57. Correia B, Fernandes J, Botica MJ, Ferreira C, Quintas A. Novel psychoactive substances: The razor's edge between therapeutical potential and psychoactive recreational misuse. *Medicines.* 2022 Mar 1;9(3):19.

9

Concluding Remarks

Kristina Adorjan, Sharon L. Walsh, and Thomas G. Schulze

The global proliferation of new psychoactive substances (NPS) over the past two decades represents a complex and rapidly evolving public health challenge. These substances, intentionally designed to mimic the effects of traditional illicit drugs while circumventing existing legal frameworks, pose significant risks due to their unregulated production, unknown potency, and unpredictable toxicity profiles. As delineated across this work, NPS encompass a broad spectrum of pharmacological classes—including synthetic cannabinoids, stimulants, hallucinogens, and depressants—each associated with distinct and often severe acute and chronic health consequences.

From a **systematic and biochemical perspective**, the diversity of NPS reflects both structural innovation and strategic manipulation of molecular targets. Their detection requires sophisticated analytical tools beyond standard immunoassays, such as high-resolution mass spectrometry and nuclear magnetic resonance, to track emerging compounds and understand their interaction with neural receptors.[1,2] These insights are vital not only for forensic identification but also for shaping effective regulation and clinical management strategies.

Stimulant NPS such as synthetic cathinones and amphetamine derivatives demonstrate profound neuropsychiatric and cardiovascular toxicity, with increasing incidence of emergency hospitalizations linked to their use. Their widespread availability via online platforms and misperceptions of legality or safety exacerbate the harm potential, particularly among youth and marginalized populations.[3,4] Similarly, **synthetic cannabinoid receptor agonists (SCRAs)** have proven especially hazardous due to their high binding affinities and potent agonist effects, leading to acute toxic effects such as seizures, psychosis, and multi-organ dysfunction.[5,6]

Hallucinogenic NPS (HNPS) mimic classical psychedelics but often display more potent and unpredictable effects. Particularly concerning are compounds like NBOMes, which have been linked to fatalities even at low doses, due to their strong serotonergic and sympathomimetic activity. The psychological risks—ranging from panic and psychosis to hallucinogen persisting perception disorder—warrant a nuanced harm-reduction approach and improved clinical awareness.[7,8]

Among the most lethal are **synthetic opioids**, particularly fentanyl analogues and emerging compounds like nitazenes, which have driven a surge in overdose deaths globally. Their extreme potency and inconsistent distribution in street drugs challenge traditional overdose-management protocols and may necessitate higher naloxone dosages and novel interventions.[9,10]

Furthermore, **vulnerable populations**—including adolescents, incarcerated individuals, and women—are disproportionately affected by NPS due to biological susceptibility, psychosocial pressures, and structural inequities. NPS use in these groups is associated with heightened risks of psychiatric comorbidity, infectious disease transmission, and systemic health deterioration. These findings highlight the urgent need for gender-responsive, trauma-informed, and context-specific interventions.[11,12]

In summary, the growing diversity, accessibility, and harm potential of NPS demand a multidisciplinary response encompassing:

- Enhanced **surveillance** and **analytical capacity** for rapid identification of new compounds;
- Rigorous **clinical research** to assess toxicity and develop treatment protocols;
- Comprehensive **public health education** to debunk myths and prevent misuse;
- Tailored **policy and harm-reduction strategies** for high-risk populations.

Without sustained international collaboration, evidence-based policy-making, and adaptive health services, the societal and medical burden of NPS will continue to escalate.

References

1. EMCDDA. *European Drug Report 2023: Trends and Developments.* European Monitoring Centre for Drugs and Drug Addiction. 2023.
2. Zawilska JB, Andrzejczak D. Next generation of novel psychoactive substances on the horizon: A complex problem to face. *Drug Alcohol Depend.* 2015;157:1–17.
3. UNODC. *World Drug Report 2022.* United Nations Office on Drugs and Crime; 2022.

4. Orsolini L, Papanti D, Corkery JM, Schifano F. Novel psychoactive substances (NPS) use in children and adolescents: Clinical features, therapeutic challenges, and emerging issues. *Curr Neuropharmacol.* 2021;19(12):2102–2124.
5. Hermanns-Clausen M, Kneisel S, Szabo B, Auwärter V. Acute toxicity due to the confirmed consumption of synthetic cannabinoids: clinical and laboratory findings. *Addiction.* 2013;108(3):534–544.
6. Castaneto MS, Gorelick DA, Desrosiers NA, Hartman RL, Pirard S, Huestis MA. Synthetic cannabinoids: Epidemiology, pharmacodynamics, and clinical implications. *Drug Alcohol Depend.* 2014;144:12–41.
7. Halberstadt AL, Geyer MA. Multiple receptors contribute to the behavioral effects of indoleamine hallucinogens. *Neuropharmacology.* 2011;61(3):364–381.
8. Lawn W, Barratt MJ, Williams M, Horne A, Winstock AR, Ling S. The NBOMe hallucinogenic drug series: Patterns of use, characteristics of users and self-reported effects. *J Psychopharmacol.* 2019;33(9):1115–1122.
9. Piper BJ, Shah DT, Simoyan OM, McCall KL, Nichols SD. Trends in medical use of opioids in the U.S., 2006–2016. *Am J Prevent Med.* 2021;60(6):756–762.
10. Scholl L, Seth P, Kariisa M, Wilson N, Baldwin G. Drug and opioid-involved overdose deaths: United States, 2013–2017. *MMWR.* 2019;67(5152):1419–1427.
11. Evans-Brown M, Sedefov R. Responding to new psychoactive substances in the European Union: Early warning, risk assessment, and control measures. *Handb Clin Neurol.* 2018;158:179–190.
12. Vento AE, Orsolini L, Vellante F, et al. Gender-related psychopathological features and comorbidities in opioid use disorder. *Front Psychiatry.* 2020;11:685.

Index

For the benefit of digital users, indexed terms that span two pages (e.g., 52–53) may, on occasion, appear on only one of those pages.

Tables, figures, and boxes are indicated by an italic *t*, *f*, and *b* following the page number.